Spinal Cord Injury: Impact and Coping

KU-319-968

Clive A. Glass

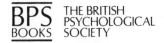

BPS BOOKS THE BRITISH PSYCHOLOGICAL SOCIETY

First published in 1999 by BPS Books (The British Psychological Society), St Andrews House, 48 Princess Road East, Leicester LE1 7DR, UK.

A catalogue record for this book is available from the British Library.

ISBN 1 85433 301 1

Typeset by Words & Graphics Ltd., Anstey, Leicestershire, UK
Printed in Great Britain by Antony Rowe Ltd., Reading, Berks

Spinal Cord Injury:
Impact and Coping

For
Stan and Joan Glass

Contents

Illustrations

Acknowledgements

This book summarizes my experiences with over 4,000 people whose lives have been affected by a spinal cord injury. It is impossible to list them all but to each I offer my thanks and appreciation for sharing their time and thoughts with me.

My views are also significantly influenced by my colleagues, past and present, and those with whom I have collaborated in Southport and throughout the world. Thank you. Many made content suggestions and read the numerous drafts and their comments are incorporated in the final text; particular thanks to Jenny, Krish, Glynn, Barbara, Bakul, Pradip, John, Julie, Suzie, Keith, Nancy, Michael and Ann.

Thanks also to Jon, the reviewers, and all the staff at the BPS for their constructive comments, patience and support.

And finally, to all my family, but with particular love and thanks to my wife Judy who was full of praise and encouragement when it mattered, proof-read and was critical when I needed it, and kept Greebo at bay from playing on the computer keys.

Copyright Acknowledgements

Preface

The experience of spinal cord injury (SCI) is one of the most devastating injuries which might affect an individual. The resultant disability, after which normal cognitive function and intellectual ability usually remains, produces not only an inability to move and feel limbs, but also the inability to control the function of internal organs and even, in severe cases, the ability to breathe independently. Eventual successful outcome following trauma is evidenced by the extent of emotional adjustment and requires more of the clinician than just an understanding of the physical impact of injury to the spinal cord.

This book is designed primarily to help recently qualified staff and professionals from all disciplines develop insight into the implications of a spinal cord injury and the role that they play in enabling the patient and their family to tolerate the complex and time consuming process of care and rehabilitation. It is aimed to have relevance not only for those who work full time in the area, but also for those (such as general practitioners) who may meet with people with spinal cord injuries less frequently; indeed those in primary care may be considered of particular importance for this client group as they act as key personnel in maintaining community well-being.

Despite the need to justify intervention with theory it is hoped the book will also provide some support to those newly injured and their families. It contains a series of quotes from injured people, their relatives and care staff to highlight the problems often faced. These have been modified only to ensure confidentiality and anonymity and their inclusion may help those newly injured to place their own reactions into context.

The book contains seven chapters. Chapter 1 addresses the morphology of the spine and spinal cord, explores the methods by which the extent of trauma may be assessed, and the common risk factors following trauma to the spinal cord. This chapter is lengthy but it is imperative that each of the complications of injury is addressed if the notion that spinal cord injury 'means you can't move arms or legs' is to be dispelled. Establishing good clinical practice for the avoidance and treatment of these physical complications is essential for promotion of optimal rehabilitation. Chapter 2 is designed to introduce the reader to the difficult area of how and when to break news. The aim of the chapter is not only to provide some pointers to good clinical practice but also to encourage the reader to reflect on their perceptions of how it might feel to be the recipient of such information. Chapter 3 critically examines those variables associated with coping and adaptation strategies adopted by individuals and families following spinal cord injury and highlights methods of intervention which have been found effective for patients, carers and staff during the immediate phase of treatment. Chapter 4 defines those issues of importance for the injured person in returning home, and how safety of the environment may be assessed. Chapter 5 addresses the importance of sexual behaviour and sexuality. It provides an information framework from which those who do wish to explore the issue further may make further inquiry.

While it is recognized that there is no such thing as an 'acceptable' level of spinal cord injury, most people living with such disability accept that tetraplegia (paralysis below the neck) is probably the most devastating experience as it produces total, usually sudden, loss of control of life. Chapter 6 therefore explores the impact of such an all encompassing injury on the individual and their family and explores the implications of returning home for all concerned.

Throughout the past 50 years there has been considerable growth in understanding, treatment and support of the effects of spinal cord injury. The final chapter of the book summarizes the current and potential developments in the care and quality of life improvement for those with SCI, and which may influence their lives in the new millennium.

As the book reflects on the author's experiences, there is an understandable bias towards exploration of the impact of spinal cord injury and care provision within the United Kingdom. However, the majority of the book, drawing heavily on the personal experiences of injured people themselves, illustrates a number of principles and concerns which encompass and have relevance within all care systems.

1

An Introduction to Spinal Cord Injury

Introduction

For those with a professional or personal interest in spinal cord injury (SCI) it is important to develop an understanding of the intrinsic physiological changes which occur following trauma to the spinal cord. Unless such changes are addressed in a timely and appropriate manner comprehensive rehabilitation may, at best, be delayed but may, at worst, result in further trauma and even death. This statement is not made with the intention to shock, simply to state an unpleasant truth. While spinal cord injury may be considered a low incidence condition, it represents a high risk and often high cost management concern.

The purpose of this first chapter is to address the morphology of the spine and spinal cord, explore the methods by which the extent of trauma may be assessed, and the common risk factors following trauma to the spinal cord. This chapter is lengthy, but it is imperative each of the complications of injury are addressed if the notion that spinal cord injury *'means you can't move arms or legs'* is to be dispelled. Establishing good clinical practice for the avoidance and treatment of these physical complications is essential for promotion of optimal rehabilitation. The emphasis for clinicians of all disciplines must always be to support the person with the injury to take control of their situation; once they leave their host spinal injuries centre their self-motivation is imperative for their long-term safety and survival.

Development of Regional Centres

Towards the latter part of the Second World War clinicians had begun to realize that specialized centres were essential to ensure the best possible recovery and rehabilitation of spinal cord injuries. Until this time it was rare for people to survive the initial trauma, with mortality rates as high as 80 per cent (Stover and Fine, 1986). It had been the discovery of pharmaceutical agents, such as the development of antibiotic therapy, which laid the foundation for improvement of mortality. However, it was the vision of a small number of clinicians, most notably Ludwig Guttmann, which enabled Great Britain to pioneer the system of total care to be available immediately after injury as well as a continuing process throughout the disabled person's life. The centres which developed were located in such a manner that every part of the country had its own 'regional' centre, with Stoke Mandeville, Warrington (later to move to Southport) on Merseyside and Sheffield promoting the initial impetus for such care. Initial admissions were the victims of battle injuries experienced during the Second World War; the notion of spinal cord injury being essentially a trauma associated with young men was thus established from this point.

While USA data indicate the average age at point of trauma as 25, the most common age at injury being 19, there is a considerable group of patients who are older at the time of injury and indeed a significant incidence among children. Trauma and disease tend not to be age specific. The notion of young reckless men being more likely to experience traumatic brain and spinal injury may simply reflect cultural, demographic and activity statistics. The age at which injury or disease occurs and the length of time for which the trauma has been experienced both appear to have some effect on adjustment and outcome. By the time they reach adolescence, children who develop renal failure are often more pessimistic concerning their future than other adolescents (Holmes, 1986). Those aged over 50 at the time they experience spinal injury often adjust less well, which may relate to the decrease in social support networks associated with age and reduction in general physical ability (Whiteneck *et al.*,1992); and patients' perceptions of disease does alter over time (Johnston *et al.*, 1990).

Perceptions of trauma do appear to be influenced by the appropriateness of an injury or disease at specific ages. The term 'tragic and untimely' is often used to explain feelings towards the injury of a young child or terminal illness in an adolescent (Owens and Naylor, 1989), while older people who die from MS or who are left severely disabled as the result of a road traffic accident are often considered at least to 'have had a good innings'. Such global oversimplifications tend to be used by relatives, and indeed staff, as coping mechanisms. There is no more acceptable time for an individual to experience an illness or disability than any other, and all parties need to develop some awareness and acceptance of personal feelings associated with such changes.

The complications of injury in older people and the admission policy of some hospitals serves to under-represent the true incidence of spinal trauma in older age groups. Changes have also occurred in patterns of survival, most notably the number of those with high tetraplegia surviving as a consequence of improved accident site paramedic care and hospital-based respiratory care systems (Heinemann *et al.*, 1989). Numerous examples exist of patients who have had road accidents where a nurse, doctor and even ambulances have been following immediately behind, witnessed the incident and provided immediate support. While patients often have little recollection of the incident, they later express their incredulity given the low probability of such a scenario.

There exist, throughout Europe and the United States, a number of specialist centres which treat and rehabilitate those who experience spinal cord injuries. In the United Kingdom there are 11 centres which take injuries from their surrounding Health Regions (see Figure 1.1).

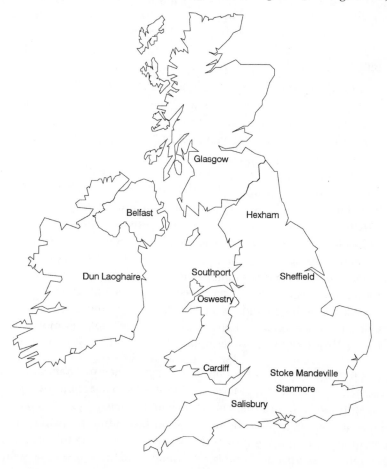

Figure 1.1: Location of spinal injuries centres in the United Kingdom.

Benefits of Rapid Transfer to SCI centres

SCI centres provide comprehensive care and rehabilitation in this highly specialized field of spinal medicine and rehabilitation. While a number of local hospitals may employ surgeons who are skilled in spinal surgery, it has long been considered that such treatment in isolation from the ability to treat the complications of the trauma is poorly founded. Although a small number of cases will understandably not be transferred due to medical complications, it is still the case that a large number of spinal trauma cases will often be delayed in their transfer to one of the specialist centres due to the well-meaning but misplaced treatment intentions of local hospitals. Such confusion among referring hospitals may be partly explained by the lack of a consistent policy concerning the availability of intensive care facilities for the acute phase of spinal trauma care. These facilities are not widely available across the United Kingdom, although a number of centres do have dedicated intensive care (IC) facilities on site, with others in the process of establishing such a facility. Check with your closest centre. A number of other centres have access to IC facilities in their host hospitals. While there is limited research into how such delays produce considerable disruption of the rehabilitation process once transfer is eventually effected, there is substantial evidence concerning the need for transfer to specialist centres on medical and rehabilitation grounds (Donovan *et al.*, 1984; Yarkony *et al.*, 1985).

Nurses treated me purely as an immobile patient rather than spinally injured; they don't realize that a red mark may be a permanent skin change ... it's not their fault, they were never taught it. Nurse training in a general hospital gives you not a single day on spinal injury [the speaker was RCN trained and a nurse tutor prior to injury]. *I would have to say it's the same in the community, unless their Authority have given them special training because of the patients they've got or they've researched it themselves they would never know. The trouble is they don't know there's a need to know and that is crucial.* (Female, 39, lower thoracic injury)

Despite the availability of evidence to support the importance of rapid transfer to a specialist spinal centre, there remain a significant number of hospital consultants who consider their specialism qualifies them to deal with the entirety of the needs of an individual following spinal cord injury. Unfortunately it is the patient who tends to suffer from such misplaced idealism, and is often referred late to such centres with considerable avoidable complications.

Joe had been treated in a local hospital following a car crash. His family repeatedly asked the consultant in charge to refer him to his Regional Spinal Injuries Centre, which was refused. As a consequence of failure of the staff to understand his care needs he developed a pressure sore which almost resulted in his death. He is now involved in separate litigation against this hospital for their contributory negligence. (Solicitor acting on behalf of male, 48, C7 complete)

Estimating the incidence and prevalence is therefore problematic, and further complicated as traumatic spinal cord injury is not a notifiable condition. Current estimates for the USA indicate an incidence of 8–10,000 new cases each year, with almost 250,000 people living with spinal cord injury (Lasfargues *et al.*, 1995). Within the UK no reliable central statistical records office exists. From the author's experience an approximate figure of 1,200 new cases each year is likely. This includes approximately 1,000 who are treated within the 10 specialist centres and a further 20 per cent who are treated less optimally by general medical and orthopaedic specialists. Of the 11 Centres across the United Kingdom which specialize in the treatment and rehabilitation of spinal cord injury there is considerable variability in the time taken to effect admission.

The Structure of the Spine and Spinal Cord

The spinal cord is an extension of the brain and runs through the centre of the backbone and is therefore protected by it. The backbone – the spine – is made up of a 33 individual bones (vertebrae) like links in a chain. These are held in place by special joints strengthened by ligaments and tough fibrous tissue. Strong muscles provide further protection to the entire length of the vertebral column. The bones which make up the spinal column are divided into four main parts:

The **CERVICAL** area (neck)	consisting of **7 vertebrae.**
The **THORACIC** area (chest)	consisting of **12 vertebrae.**
The **LUMBAR** area (low back)	consisting of **5 vertebrae.**
The **SACRAL** area (lower back)	consisting of **5 fused vertebrae.**
The **COCCYGEAL** area (the 'tail' of the spine)	consisting of **4 fused vertebrae.**

The five vertebrae that constitute the sacral region are fused together and in effect are represented by one triangular bone – the sacrum – and the remaining four vertebrae are very small – the coccyx – and of no real consequence in human beings. The extension of this segment into several vertebrae forms the tail in animals.

In total there are 31 pairs of spinal nerve roots which generally leave the cord below the corresponding vertebral level. However, as the spinal cord is shorter than the spinal column the lumbar and sacral nerves have long roots which together are called the 'cauda equina' (or horse's tail). At the level of the last two thoracic nerve segments the cord becomes smaller and is called the conus medullaris.

Each spinal cord nerve segment communicates with specific parts of the body through spinal nerves. Sensory fibres from each spinal nerve serve a particular surface (dermatome) of the skin. This is illustrated by Figure 1.2.

The spinal cord operates essentially as a communications network, in that messages are passed down the cord from the brain to every

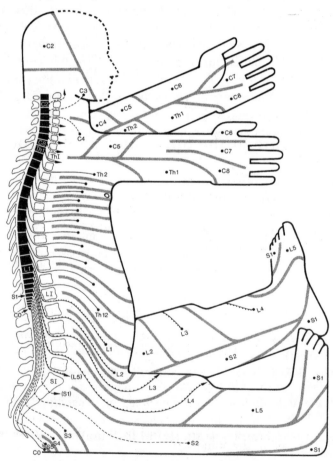

Figure 1.2: Relationship of spinal column to cord segments, nerve roots and dermatones (reproduced from Mumenthaler, 1985).

6

part of the body. Messages also travel up through the spinal cord to inform the brain; in order to lift a leg the brain sends a nerve impulse down the spinal cord to a spinal nerve which then sends the message on to the specific muscle (the motor pathway). Similarly, the ability to feel when someone touches the hand or foot depends on impulses travelling from the skin, through the spinal nerve, up through the spinal cord and on to the brain (the sensory pathway). It would be wrong, however, to think of the spinal cord as a bundle of cables; the grey matter of the cord is essentially a thick, viscous material containing innumerable neurones and their associated communicating dendrites and axons. Running through the length of this cord is a central canal which contains cerebro-spinal fluid. If a cross-section of the spinal cord is examined, the central portion (grey matter) comprises the anterior, lateral and posterior horns. Essentially these three areas contain three different types of cells: the anterior horn contains lower motor neurones whose axons terminate in skeletal muscles, the lateral horns contain cells that give rise to sympathetic fibres of the autonomic nervous system and the posterior horns contain sensory fibres. The white matter surrounding the grey matter contains the afferent and efferent tracts that conduct impulses from the cortex and to and from the brainstem and cerebellum. The spinal cord therefore not only transmits messages (impulses) but also contains a central core of nerve cells that mediates various functions and reflexes (see Figures 1.3a and 1.3b).

Damage to the Spinal Cord

Trauma to the spinal cord may be developmental or acquired. Developmental traumas include spina bifida, scoliosis, spondylolisthesis and familial paralysis. Acquired traumas to the spinal cord arise out of a number of situations.

> *I went to bed just feeling a bit under the weather. I woke at about four and remember sweating a great deal. I drank some water and drifted back to sleep. When I woke up I felt weak but put it down to 'flu. It was only as the day went on that I realized something was going on. I couldn't get out of bed to go to the bathroom and when my wife and son tried to stand me I couldn't take the weight. I've been in the wheelchair ever since.* (Male, 48, mid-thoracic paraplegia after viral infection)

Infections to the spinal cord arising out of bacterial or viral infection produce particular problems of adjustment – one moment the person

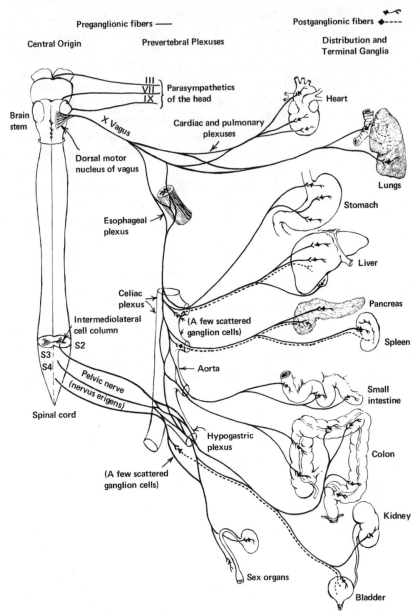

Figure 1.3a: The parasympathetic nervous system
(reproduced from Barr and Kiernan, 1983).

is fine, the next they are left with varying degrees of disability. Their adjustment is complicated by the uncertainty of further improvement or deterioration.

Others experience degenerative conditions, such as spondylosis or disc herniation; neurological degeneration resulting in multiple sclerosis and motor neurone disease (amyotrophic lateral sclerosis); neoplasms (benign or malignant cancers), which are a more common

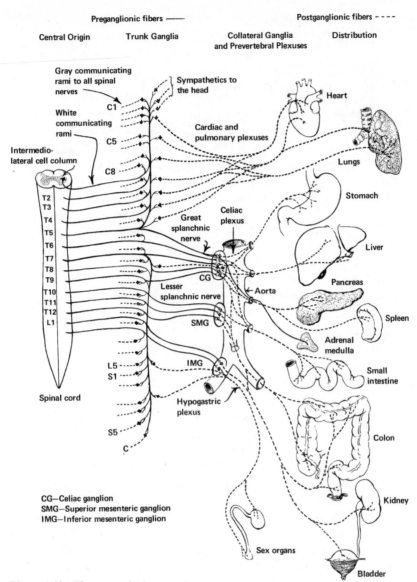

Figure 1.3b: The sympathetic nervous system
(reproduced from Barr and Kiernan, 1983).

cause of spinal cord damage than traumatic injury (Staas *et al.*, 1988); vascular insults such as aneurysm, embolism and spontaneous anterior artery thrombosis; and some as indirect insult associated with the treatment of other conditions, such as through radiation, surgery or vaccination.

Whatever the cause, the resultant spinal cord injury and associated levels of disability present a considerable challenge not only to the injured person but to their family and friends, care staff and the community in general. An awareness of physiology and morphology is an important precursor to developing a wider understanding of the complexities of adjustment.

Prevalence and Incidence of SCI

Prevalence, or the total number, of traumatic spinal cord injuries in the UK is estimated to be approximately 25,000. Taking into account those with non-traumatic spinal cord injury this figure would be closer to 40,000. The vast majority of injuries remain the result of motor vehicle accidents. However a further significant percentage of injuries (17 per cent) arise out of falls within the home. A comparison of aetiology for the UK and USA is highlighted in Table 1.1 (derived from web page publication by the UK Spinal Injuries Association (1998); American Spinal Injuries Association, 1997).

In the USA (Parsons and Lamertse, 1991) it is estimated that the incidence of non-traumatic spinal cord injury is comparable to that of traumatic injuries, while in the UK the estimate of the Spinal Injuries Association is 16 per cent (Spinal Injuries Association, 1992).

Principal Effects of SCI: (1) Defining the Loss

So what happens if the spinal cord is damaged either by injury associated with fracture and/or dislocation of the vertebrae or by various other causes? Considering that the basic function of the spinal cord is transmission of messages between the brain and the rest of the body, any interruption of the 'cabling' will isolate the portion of the body below the level of the break, from central (conscious) control and perception. Therefore if the person wants to move a part of the body below the break, the message from the brain will not get through and no movement will be possible. Conversely, if the person is touched below the level of the break the message will not be able to reach the brain and they will not be able to appreciate the touch.

The inability to 'feel' also includes the inability to perceive temperature changes and, more importantly, the inability to perceive an image of the body in space. Those with SCI are often not able to be sure in which position their limbs below the break are being placed or, indeed, exactly where they are.

When I was first injured [C4, complete tetraplegia] *I got all sorts of strange messages like my feet were floating and my legs were crossed. When I could sit up and see them it wasn't as bad and now I think I have a good awareness of where my body is. I still*

Table 1.1: *Comparison of USA and UK spinal cord injury incidence, causes and resultant neurological level.*

	USA		UK	
Population	243.75 million		58 million	
Incidence	7,800 injuries per year		1,100 injuries per year	
Relative incidence	32 injuries/ per million/pa		19 injuries/ per million/pa	
Cause of injury	**n**	**%**	**n**	**%**
RTA	3,432	44	660	60
Violence	1,872	24	11	1
Fall	1,716	22	187	17
Sport	624	8	220	20
Other	156	2	22	2
Level of injury				
Tetraplegia	4,134	53	660	60
(of which) C4 above	413	10	66	10
C5	579	14	66	10
C6 and C7	3,142	76	528	80
Paraplegia				
(of which) T1–7	1,246	34	176	40
T8–10	1,136	31	110	25
T11–L1	917	25	88	20
L1 and below	367	10	66	15

feel insecure on occasions when they first sit me in the chair ... sometimes just being able to move my neck makes me feel like I'm a head on top of a lump of meat. (Male, 21, C4 complete tetraplegia)

All these changes are part of the general term 'paralysis', which in itself contains two main features.

Level of Injury

This denotes the exact level of the damage to the spinal cord and is expressed as C5, T4, T10, L1, etc. This is the level below which power and/or sensation have been affected. The level of impairment experienced by an individual may be assessed by examining the relative extent of sensory and motor damage. Systematic examination of sensory and motor perception along the entire spinal cord enables an assessment to be made of the level and extent of spinal cord injury. As the neurological level of injury may not equate to the level of injury to the vertebra it is common to report the degree of injury as the lowest level at which normal sensory and motor power is maintained on both sides of the body. Defining the level at which the injured person has retained power and sensation is of greatest relevance to functional goals and likely eventual level of independence.

Comprehensive motor and sensory examination is therefore imperative and the system promoted by the American Spinal Injury Association (ASIA, 1992) is notable in this respect. Motor examination involves testing a key muscle (one on both the right and left sides of the body) in 10 paired myotomes (a group of muscle fibres innervated by a single spinal segment). These paired myotomes were selected in the development of the ASIA scale because of their consistency of being innervated by specific spinal segments (C5–T1 and L2–S1 inclusive). Similarly, sensory examination requires assessment of 28 dermatomes (an area of skin innervated by sensory axons from one spinal root) to light touch and pinprick on the right and left hand sides of the body (see Figure 1.4).

Extent of Paralysis

This is described as 'complete' or 'incomplete' depending on the extent to which power and sensation are affected. If, for example, the injury or damage to the spinal cord is described as complete below T4, it is meant to indicate that below the level of the nipples there is total abolition of power and sensation. It must also be noted that, dependent upon the level of injury, all bodily function may be compromised.

When either the motor or sensory pathway is interrupted, or usually both, as occurs after a spinal injury, the result is paralysis and a lack of sensation. The amount of loss of sensation and paralysis that occurs depends upon the site of the injury and the extent of damage to the spinal cord. The overall functional effects of complete spinal cord injuries at specific levels are shown in Table 1.2.

Not all spinal cord injuries may be considered 'complete'. The term 'incomplete', however, is very vague and all it is meant to indicate is that the individual is not totally deprived of power and sensation; involvement of power and sensation may not, for example, be symmetrical. In certain cases people experience trauma to the central portion of the cord which frequently results in good lower limb

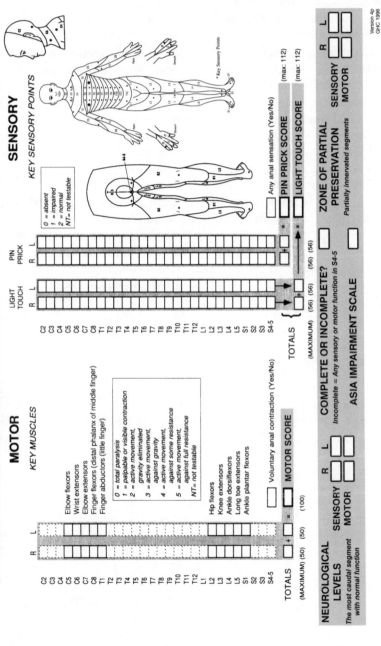

Figure 1.4: Standard neurological classification of spinal injury: ASIA scale (reproduced from International Standards for Neurological and Functional Classification of Spinal Cord Injury, 1996).

Table 1.2: Functional abilities associated with complete level of spinal cord injury.

Neurological level	Muscles remaining under control	Functional goals
C1–3	Limited neck control	Respiratory function dependent on mechanical ventilation or phrenic nerve stimulators. Electric wheelchair mobility, mouthstick, infrared control/ other interface activities, page turner, environmental controls, typewriter, computer.
C4	Neck control scapular elevators	Electric wheelchair mobility. Limited feeding possible with ball bearing feeders, mouthstick, infrared/other interface activities, page turner, typewriter, computer, environmental control.
C5	Deltoids, fair to good shoulders, bicepts, elbow flexion	Manual wheelchair adapted rims; short distances and smooth surfaces. Electric wheelchair for outside or long distances. Assistance needed with transfers. May be able to relieve pressure. Self-feeding with splints, operate typewriter, telephone, computer, etc., with assistive devices.
C6	Dorsiflexion, wrist extension	Able to propel wheelchair but may need electric wheelchair for long distances. Sliding board transfers often without assistance. Able to feel self with assistive device, bathe and dress upper half but may need assistance with lower half. Drive with hand controls and able to write with splints.

Neurological level	Muscles remaining under control	Functional goals
C7–8	Weak shoulder depression, weak triceps, elbow extension, finger flexion, extension, and abduction	Independent with transfers, feeding, bathing and bowel and bladder care. May need assistance with floor to chair transfers. Able to drive with hand controls.
T1–2	Intrinsics	Fine motor skills involving fingers.
T3–10	Intact upper extremities. Partial to good trunk balance	Fully independent in wheelchair skills including ramps and kerbs. Independent in all transfers. Able to drive with hand controls.
T12–L2	Hip flexors	Ability to stand and move for few steps/distance with long leg orthoses and crutches. May ambulate short distances in home with long leg orthoses and crutches.
L2–4	Hip abductors	Stand and walk with short leg orthoses (with or without crutches).
L5–S3	Movement of ankles and toes	Stand and walk without assistive devices.
S2–4	Perineal musculature bowel, bladder, sex organs. Movement of large toe	Management of elimination through specific bowel and bladder programmes.

NB: Every injury is different; therefore functional goals should be viewed only as general guidlelines

function but reduced upper limb and hand function; others may experience good power but limited sensation to one side of the body and the converse to the other side. This arises due to the fact that injury to the spinal cord (which is a combination of actual physical injury to nerve cells or fibres and 'indirect' damage to these structures due to disruption of blood supply) is not always clearly in a sharp line across the cord and may be in an irregular pattern, extending above or below the exact site of primary injury. Injuries to specific areas of the spinal cord will therefore produce specific effects on function and well-established syndromes (see Figure 1.5).

Given the complexity of the trauma the spine may experience, it is common for staff to explain to newly injured people that the extent of their trauma is unique. Establishing a perception of the 'uniqueness' of each individual's trauma assists in two ways; it stops people developing false hope often gained through conversation with other relatives or friends who 'know of someone who did the same thing and they are walking now', and also supports a concept of 'ownership':

Knowing that the injury was unique meant I had a vested interest in exploring all the things going on in my body. (Male, 29, C6 complete tetraplegia)

It is certainly the case, however, that those with incomplete lesions experience considerable difficulties of adjustment. For those with complete trauma there is the certainty of what remains; for those with incomplete injuries the process of rehabilitation is often agonizingly slow and unpredictable, resulting in considerable frustration and frequent over-optimistic perceptions of the eventual level of ability.

It is important also to recognize that very serious spinal cord injury with paralysis may occur without any significant, demonstrable fracture or dislocation. What is of concern is the injury to the spinal cord which is the basic element in the development of the paralysis. Indeed on many occasions there can be quite substantial disruption of the vertebral column but the spinal cord may be totally spared and there may be no paralysis at all. It is not uncommon for people to limp into an accident department after a fall at home or after a traffic accident complaining of pain in the back or neck and ultimately discover there was indeed a fracture or dislocation of the spine. Ideally therefore, the term 'spinal cord injury' should be used rather than 'spinal injury'.

Immediately after the injury, there is a total lack of movement and reflexes in the affected parts which is referred to as 'spinal shock'. This stage may last for several weeks before resolution and accurate assessment of any permanent damage becomes possible. It is therefore

	MUSCLE TONE	MOTOR FUNCTION	TOUCH SENSITIVE	DEEP SENSITIVITY	TEMPERATURE SENSATION
COMPLETE TRANSVERSE SYNDROME	↑	BILATERAL +	+	+	+
BROWN-SEQUARD SYNDROME	=↑	=+	x→	=+	x+
CONUS MEDULLARIS SYNDROME	NO	NO	SADDLE ANAESTH	SADDLE ANAESTHESIA	SADDLE ANAESTHESIA
LESIONS AROUND CENTRAL CANAL	→	+	NO	NO	+
POSTERIOR COLUMN LESIONS	NO	NO	NO	+	NO
ANTERIOR HORN LESIONS	→	+	NO	NO	NO

KEY

NO	=	Normal
+	=	Affected
↑	=	Increased
↔	=	Decreased
=	=	Ipsilateral
x	=	Contralateral

Figure 1.5: Symptoms related to location of spinal cord lesion (adapted from Mumenthaler, 1985).

unwise to attempt definitive forecasts immediately after injury, particularly if there is some preservation of sensation and power of
movement. Repeated examinations are therefore necessary and these
are a regular feature of early observation and care.

There exists a classification system, developed by Hans Frankel and
his co-workers, for defining the neurological extent of spinal cord
injury (Frankel *et al.*, 1969). The ASIA scale modifies this slightly to
grade degree of impairment as follows:

A = Complete. No sensory or motor function is preserved below the neurological level.

B = Incomplete. Sensory but no motor function is
preserved below the neurological level.

C = Incomplete. Motor function is preserved below
the neurological level. The majority of key muscles
below the neurological level have a muscle
grade of less than 3.

D = Incomplete. Motor function is preserved below
the neurological level. The majority of key muscles
below the neurological level have a muscle
grade greater than or equal to 3.

E = Normal. Sensory and motor function is normal.
(Reflexes may be abnormal.)

Repair and resolution after injury varies considerably depending on
the type of tissue that is damaged. As a general principle, the more
sophisticated the tissue, the less it will heal and return to its previous
state. This is best illustrated in the case of skin. If the whole thickness
of skin is lost by injury or burn, though eventually a 'covering' is
re-established, the new skin will not be of the original texture or
colour and there will be no regeneration of hair or sweat glands.
Nervous tissue, being highly evolved, does not fully recover and
re-establish connections. Therefore, there is a high probability in many
instances the paralysis will be permanent. Recent scientific study and
research have shown that, contrary to the long-established conviction
that no regeneration at all was possible in the nervous system (except
of nerves outside the confines of the spinal cord), some limited
regeneration has indeed been shown in animal models. However, for
all practical purposes the present state of knowledge and clinical
observation do not allow any justifiable alternative than to assume
that the probability of significant recovery after major spinal cord
injury is indeed very remote.

Principal Effects of SCI: (2) Functional effects

It must be noted that disruption of the pathway of nervous connection following spinal cord injury affects not only the ability to move the limbs, but also a wide range of internal physical functions. While it is impossible to state what functional ability an individual will attain post injury, a number of internal functions are commonly affected. These include impairment of voiding from the bladder and bowels, respiratory dysfunction, impairment of sexual function (see Chapter 5), reflex sweating and thermoregulation difficulties; patients referred to specialist centres receive wide ranging rehabilitation geared towards counteracting these effects. In order that some initial understanding of the wider implications of the trauma may be addressed, the following complications are highlighted not only because of their particular importance in maintenance of life, but also because of their relevance throughout the injured person's life.

Effect on the Bladder

One of the features of injury to the spinal cord is the inability to pass urine and know when the bladder is full. There are a number of methods of achieving drainage dependant on the nature of the spinal cord injury. Initial management during the period of 'spinal shock' for both men and women is normally by catheterization, whereby a small plastic tube is inserted into the bladder. It may be introduced through the urethra and removed after the bladder has been emptied and the procedure repeated at regular intervals (intermittent catheterization) or it may be left in the bladder and attached to a plastic bag which, while an in patient, hangs on the side of the bed or is attached to the leg with a strap once mobilization occurs (continuous catheterization). The urine drains away into this bag which can be emptied, or measured and recorded at times of need.

On occasions the catheter may be introduced through the abdominal wall, just above the pubic bone. This procedure is called 'suprapubic catheterization'. The bladder will then be on continuous drainage.

After the phase of 'spinal shock', there are several possible outcomes and every one of these has its own specific mode of management, depending on the nature and extent of the spinal cord damage.

If the damage to the cord is only mild, although in the early stage there may be need for catheterization, the bladder may recover. Even where moderate weakness in the muscles of the limbs may persist, the bladder could escape from being substantially affected. The person may then get back to the situation which existed prior to injury. In men some form of external collecting device may be necessary when out for any length of time, and while at home, particularly at night, it may be necessary to have a urine bottle handy. For women, a strict drill of keeping the bladder small by regular emptying would be necessary. Such a happy outcome, however, is not common and the recovery may be only partial.

If the damage to the cord is substantial, neurological control of the bladder will be impaired resulting in what is generally called a 'neuropathic bladder'. There are essentially two types of neuropathic bladder that can result from spinal cord damage.

Supra sacral bladder (also called 'reflex bladder')

Disruption of nervous pathways in the spinal cord results in the brain no longer being able to influence control over the urinary bladder. In supra sacral bladders, the segments of the cord that control bladder activity and the nerves that carry the messages from the cord to the bladder are intact and the bladder can, therefore, develop its own pattern of activity. As the segments in the spinal cord that control bladder activity (S2, 3, 4) are intact, messages from the bladder, transmitted through its nerve fibres, will be received and processed by the spinal cord segments which will act as the highest level of control (as the brain no longer controls as it did before the injury). The message to contract the bladder will go down through nerve fibres to the bladder and the bladder will therefore empty, but the individual will not be aware of this as the brain cannot receive any message. Sometimes the person experiences a strange feeling. If an appropriate external collecting device is not in place, the person may wet their clothes, wheelchair cushion or bed.

In men some form of a sheath is put over the penis and connected to a 'leg bag'. In women a catheter has been the only real choice, which also connects to a bag held in place on the leg, underneath a skirt or trousers. The other alternative is pads, which women often find act as an irritant to skin, and are functionally cumbersome, inconvenient and socially unacceptable. At night a larger volume drainage bag is often used in order not to disturb sleep. It remains important for all patients to drink a reasonable amount of fluid as too concentrated urine is inclined to form crystals and block catheters.

Voiding is rarely a problem in women due to the relative absence of resistance (which in men is determined by the prostate gland) and short length of the urethra. On occasions where there is some relative outlet obstruction, simple urethral dilatation may be all that is required. In men, on many occasions, even if the bladder has indeed the ability to contract (reflex bladder) it may not be possible to empty it adequately. Such a situation has a rather complicated sounding name – 'detrusor–sphincter dyssynergia'. It means that the detrusor (the muscle fibres of the bladder) and the sphincter (the outlet of the bladder) are not working in co-ordination with each other. A bladder that is inadequately emptied is vulnerable to infection and there are essentially four ways in which this may be resolved:

1. Treatment with drugs.
2. Re-establishing catheter drainage.
3. Surgical operations on the bladder outlet to redress the imbalance of activity between detrusor and sphincter.
4. Implanting radio frequency controlled stimulators in the spinal cord.

Sacral bladder (also called 'lower motor neurone bladder')

If the sacral segments (S2, 3, 4) or the nerves that carry the messages from these segments to the bladder are damaged (sometimes this can occur even if the main site of damage to the spinal cord is much higher), a 'reflex' bladder cannot develop as there is no 'centre' in the cord which can either respond to messages that are received from the bladder or initiate contraction of the bladder by sending messages down (the brain, of course, remains without any control). The part of the nervous mechanism from the brain to the level of the spinal cord is called the 'upper motor neurone' and from the cord down to the target organ, the bladder, is called the 'lower motor neurone'. Hence the name, 'lower motor neurone bladder'.

If the bladder has lost its inherent ability to contract, the only way in which it can be emptied is by straining hard to squeeze urine out of the bladder or by catheterization. Straining is an unreliable method as it is not always possible to be sure the bladder is completely empty. The only reliable method therefore is catheterization.

Effect on the Bowels

Spinal cord injury also affects bowel control and patients in specialist centres are taught a strict regime to ensure adequate movement. In the early stages of the injury patients are not able to open their bowels and it is done by manual evacuation. This is done by inserting suppositories or rectal solution and a short while later the nurse inserts a gloved finger into the rectum and removes the faeces. Patients understandably feel embarrassed and considerable emotional support is required at this time to enable each person to overcome this problem. Long-term management depends on the level of damage, particularly how much the person can physically manage on their own and how much help is needed from others.

Sensory and motor examinations can be used to determine the

extent of alteration of bowel function. The bowel may be affected in two ways. It may no longer be under the control of higher cortical centres but retains reflex function (reflex neurogenic bowel) which means it will empty in response to the build up of faeces. In this case the aim of intervention is to develop a predictable pattern of voiding so that toileting may be planned and accidents kept to a minimum. The bowel may also be disrupted due to damage to the sacral nerves (S2–4) such that reflex voiding is disrupted. In this case although incontinence remains a problem there may also be difficulties due to retention.

Eventually most people are established on a regime where they have total control over when and where they open their bowels. Establishing an acceptable bowel management regime is imperative for determining subsequent quality of life; the social inconvenience and embarrassment associated with bowel 'accidents' must be avoided at all costs and an appropriate dietary regime is essential.

Effect on Breathing

If the damage to the spinal cord involves the thoracic segments there will be varying degrees of respiratory inadequacy depending on the site of damage. Reduction of vital capacity will mean the person may have difficulty in coughing and speaking loudly. It is often possible to increase vital capacity by taking deep breaths regularly, following a strict drill. An incentive spirometer is a useful device for providing feedback in these circumstances as it provides a visual impression of achievement.

Where vital capacity has been reduced, the person's ability to cough is usually compromised. Such people may require assistance with coughing and are also more prone to infections, mainly as they may not have the power to bring up phlegm and keep their airways clear. Simple precautions are appropriate and effective:

(a) When going out of doors wear adequate clothing and do not expose the chest to chill winds.
(b) Ensure the injured person does not smoke and that others do not smoke in their presence.
(c) Organize annual preventative injections for influenza.

For a number of people the severity of their spinal trauma is such that they require artificial support of breathing using a ventilator. In the majority of these cases this will be a temporary condition, until their trauma has stabilized, but for a significant minority this support will be a permanent feature of their lives. Issues associated with long term and permanent ventilation are addressed more fully in Chapter 6.

Effect on the skin

There are three factors that make weight bearing areas of the skin vulnerable:

1. As sensory impulses from areas of skin affected by the paralysis do not reach the brain, the person is not conscious of sensations of continued pressure, heat, cold or pain.
2. As the paralysis makes the person unable to move the affected parts of their body they are unable to adjust their position which, before the spinal cord damage, occurred automatically and as a matter of course – when changing position, crossing legs, turning in bed and various movements to eliminate pressure.
3. The skin itself has less vitality due to the reduction of blood supply as a result of inadequate autonomic control and a lowered pressure head. Maceration of skin due to leakage from bladder or bowels may make this situation worse.

From the point of trauma hospital staff initiate a regime whereby the person is turned in bed regularly every two or three hours either in a powered bed or manually. Such a precaution remains necessary when established in the wheelchair. Areas of skin subjected to continual pressure will show well-marked redness quickly progressing to blistering, swelling and breakdown. Where the surrounding tissues are thicker, repeated pressure often produces a fibrous subcutaneous tissue called a bursa. If left untreated this may cause further pressure to the skin and eventually form pressure sores. Photograph 1.1 (p. 24) shows a severe case where skin breakdown has occurred. The bursa is the large white object in the centre of the wound.

Where the bones of the body are closest to the surface, there is the greatest risk of pressure sore formation. Photograph 1.2 shows extensive sores which developed at both trochanters, ischia and anal cleft when a patient who normally mobilized for four hours was left in his chair for seven hours. To add insult to injury he was repeatedly mobilized for three more days by well-meaning care staff.

Furthermore, sores can occur in places where they may not be expected. The breakdown of skin in Photograph 1.3 occurred simply because the patient's shoes were too tight.

Avoidance of pressure sores rather than treatment

Avoidance of pressure sores is therefore essential. During the early stages of mobilization patients are taught to inspect pressure bearing

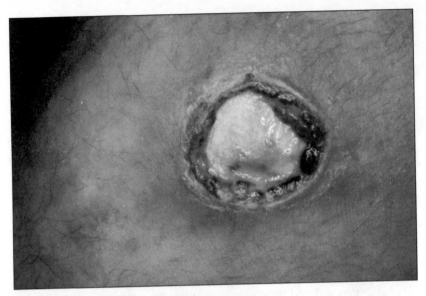

Photograph 1.1: Gluteal bursar.

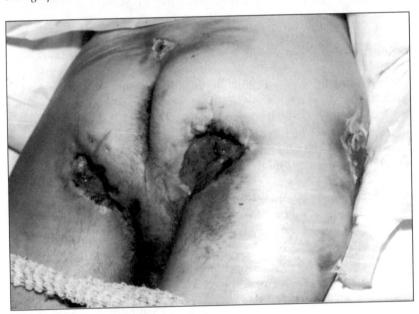

Photograph 1.2: Trochanteric, ischial and cleft pressure sores.

areas, mainly over the hips and buttocks regularly whenever they are transferred to bed from the chair to ensure there is no redness or any other warning sign of constant pressure. If there is indeed any such sign it is imperative that the person stays in bed until it has resolved. This may be very annoying and frustrating, but unless this is done the skin may rapidly deteriorate and produce a sore which will mean

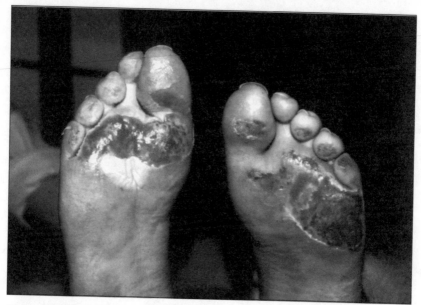

Photograph 1.3: Pressure sores to the feet.

confinement to bed again for several days, weeks or in extreme cases months.

There are simple precautions that can compensate lack of sensation and inability to move, and that all wheelchair users may learn:

- Is the outside of the ankle pressing against the metal strut of the foot rest of the wheelchair?
- Has the foot slipped forward, with the heel resting on the footplate?
- Has the cushion slipped so the person is sitting skewed, producing unequal distribution of weight, rubbing one hip on the side of the chair?

Regular lifting to relieve pressure would normally be accomplished by the patients themselves, even in cases of reduced upper limb power; those who cannot lift are often capable of tilting themselves sideways at regular intervals to relieve pressure over each buttock in turn. Those with lesions resulting in no arm or trunk control require the support of family or carers to reduce the effects of pressure.

Sores, even if they heal satisfactorily, leave scars. Scars are inelastic, and inelastic skin will break down quicker than smooth and elastic skin; therefore the occurrence of one sore makes the individual prone to a second one. Redness, which is the first and most important early warning signal, may be missed in those who have dark skin. Much greater vigilance is therefore necessary.

It is important to mention clothing in relation to the individual's potential for skin marking. What a person wears is of importance when sitting in the wheelchair, as pressure from clothing is of much relevance to the care of the skin. It is also relevant to mobility and learning how to transfer to and from the wheelchair. Track suits or other loose clothing may not always be ideal as they may crease under the legs and buttocks unnoticed. Similarly, due to increased oedema (swelling) of the ankles, socks should not be too tight; also shoe sizing initially needs much thought as this might have changed because of some swelling of the feet due to pooling of blood.

Effects of Pain

Pain is essentially the net result of sensory and emotional experience of discomfort, which is usually associated with threatened or actual physical damage or irritation (Sanders, 1985). It is common following any injury or assault to experience immediate and often severe pain. However, in certain circumstances chronic pain syndromes may develop which significantly disrupt ongoing abilities and quality of life.

> It's like someone has put a belt around my stomach and as I sit in the chair they are trying to make it tighter and tighter. I find it increasingly difficult to breathe and most days I give in after a couple of hours and have to get back into bed. I could stand it more if only I could get a good night's sleep. I look awful, I'm more irritable and everyone is getting fed up with me. (Female, 62, sensory incomplete C7 tetraplegia)

There is considerable variability in the level of incapacity which pain promotes, with some individuals able to tolerate pain beyond that which might be accepted as tolerable by others. There are essentially three components to pain perception, each of which has particular relevance for those with spinal cord injury.

1. Physiological factors, such as damage to nerve roots, deafferentation, and mechanical instability or deformity provide a physical basis.
2. Psychological factors, such as affective state disorders or acute stress, alter perceptions of these physical problems.
3. Social circumstances, which may have altered as a consequence of trauma may be more or less supportive, and involvement in litigation (Glass *et al.*, 1997b) all influence day-to-day pain tolerance.

However, one of the commonly reported difficulties which faces those with chronic pain, is the perceived lack of other people's understanding of its importance:

> *Some days June's supportive but she's not the one who's feeling it. I suppose it's written on my face when it wakes me up and that tends to set the scene for the rest of the day. I don't mean to be awful, but I'd like her to experience it for just one day. I know now how deaf people must feel.* (Male, 52, T10 complete paraplegia)

Chronic pain experienced over a long period often leads to preoccupation such that life begins to revolve around the pain, visits to doctors to attempt to treat the pain, and rituals associated with the consumption of pain medications. Given the multiplicity of factors associated with the perception of and coping with pain, effective management is best achieved through pain clinics within spinal injuries centres where a wide range of professional support can be provided in a structured approach.

(Fordyce, 1976)

Such programmes typically include:

- Reducing the patient's experience of pain.
- Supporting modifications to activities and lifestyle.
- Regulation of drug therapy and reliance on medical services.
- Promoting interpersonal skills and relationships.

Such systems of support have been shown to have considerable benefits for a wide range of chronic pain conditions following trauma. However, despite the well-accepted effects of pain following spinal cord injury, there is little systematic research undertaken in the area (Mariano, 1992). Recent attempts to quantify pain prevalence and type (Wagner Anke *et al.*, 1995) have shown the problem present in over 60 per cent of people following discharge, and some association with increased age at time of trauma and elevated psychological distress while an inpatient. Bonica (1991) undertook a review of 10 studies of pain following spinal cord injury which showed 69 per cent of patients experienced significant pain, with 30 per cent experiencing neuropathic pain. Eide (1998) used a more accurate classification for presenting pain (musculo-skeletal, visceral and neuropathic; with neuropathic pain further subdivided into peripheral and centrally mediated pain). He estimated 10–20 per cent of patients experience the most severe and difficult to treat centrally mediated neuropathic pain and proposed further research to investigate the neurochemical changes that may influence neuronal hyperactivity and pain perception.

Effect on Blood Pressure

Postural hypotension literally means reduction in the blood pressure due to erect posture. When a person first sits upright or is tilted to achieve a 'standing' posture it is common to 'feel faint', evidenced by the eyes going out of focus and feeling 'hollow' inside. Soon after they are laid down again, or if the wheelchair is fully tilted back, the person will feel normal again. Occasionally, patients also experience pronounced sweating of the face. There is a higher tendency for this to occur if the spinal cord injury is at a level of T6 or above, though it is not uncommon in people with injury below this level.

In order for the heart to pump blood to the brain against gravity, to ensure that the correct amount of blood reaches the brain after every heart beat, there must be sufficient filling up of the chambers of the heart, so that there is an adequate amount of blood to pump out. The chambers of the heart can only fill if the blood from the rest of the body (trunk and legs) is flowing back efficiently. This happens as the blood vessels in the abdomen and legs are under nervous control and retain 'tone', which is a co-ordinated and controlled ability to relax (dilate) and tighten (constrict), according to need. Such activity is severely compromised or abolished by spinal cord injury. As blood from the feet has to travel four or five feet against gravity while standing, it is fundamental that the tone is regulated so that the blood vessels do not produce pooling of blood by dilating. There are pressure sensors within the circulatory system which are extremely sensitive and mediate the necessary constriction or dilatation through the 'autonomic nervous system' to ensure there is adequate blood supply to the brain and indeed the rest of the body. When lying down, the feet, heart and the head are at the same level and the need to work against gravity is not a very crucial factor. Normally, when a person suddenly sits or stands up from a lying posture this competent and efficient system comes into operation in record time and so the brain is not denied the necessary pressure head of blood. This is the reason why people often feel faint if they stand up too quickly, and the situation is usually remedied with the age old advice of putting the head between the knees. The head and the heart will then come to be at the same level and heart will not have to work against gravity.

Although this system of co-ordination and control is situated in the spinal cord in the thoracic region, it is mediated by higher centres in the brain. If the damage to the spinal cord is at a level whereby the autonomic nervous system is isolated (out of control by the brain) due to the damage (thereby producing a barrier for conduction of nervous impulses), such an efficient adjustment becomes impossible. Blood is pooled in the legs, the chambers of the heart do not get adequately filled and consequently the brain does not receive enough blood and the person faints. As the pooling of blood is responsible for reduction in blood pressure and blood flow to the brain it may be necessary in certain cases to compensate dilatation by elastic bandages round the legs or abdominal binders. On most occasions, there will be adjustment in time. However, some vulnerability to hypotension and the need for care and attention during change of posture may remain as a permanent feature of life. When in the wheelchair, if the person begins to feel dizzy, this may be rectified by another person tilting the chair backwards until the upper body is parallel with the floor. This results in increasing the blood pressure and they will feel better quite quickly. At this time, return to the upright position may be made gradually.

Effect on Temperature Regulation

The body's temperature is also maintained by the autonomic nervous system and therefore temperature regulation is another aspect of the physiology that is often disturbed by spinal cord damage. Like pressure sensors maintaining blood pressure there are sensors that regulate temperature and abolition of their action results in the body assuming the temperature of the surrounding atmosphere.

Hypothermia refers to a decrease in body temperature. This will happen if the person is exposed to undue draught or if they do not wear adequate and appropriate clothing. It is essential that room temperature is maintained around 85 degrees Fahrenheit (approximately 32 degrees Celsius). If this is not the case then the person must move to a warmer room and use more blankets. It is important that cold areas of the body are not rubbed to make them warm as this may damage the skin. Similarly, if the person wears too many clothes or is in a room artificially heated to a high level, they may go into a state of pyrexia (increased temperature and fever). All that needs to be done to reduce this is to move them to a cooler area or remove excess clothing.

However, it is also important in this connection to note that there are several other causes for increased temperature. In the event of urinary infection, or any other form of sepsis, the temperature will increase and it is important to be aware of this inherent vulnerability before significance of the fever is assessed.

With both increased temperature and hypothermia, prevention is better than cure. With experience, each person learns how much time they are able to spend in hot or cold areas, which parts of their body are most susceptible and how to cope with sudden changes in temperature.

Effect on Autonomic Nervous System (Dysreflexia or Autonomic Hyperreflexia)

This is another result of the isolation of the autonomic nervous system and therefore is most frequently seen when the level of damage is above the main part of the outflow of the system situated in the thoracic spinal cord – above the level of T4 or 5. Even if damage is below this level dysreflexia might happen, but as the level of injury goes down the probability diminishes.

If there is any enlargement of a 'hollow' organ (e.g. urinary bladder or bowel), irritation of delicate tissue (e.g. the lining of urethra or bladder), or a variety of stimulations within the body, nervous impulses are sent up nerves that are directed towards the brain. As these impulses cannot reach the brain because of the spinal cord damage, the individual does not perceive them. However, these impulses reach the autonomic nervous system which release particular chemicals into the circulation, resulting in a sudden and intense increase in the blood pressure. There will also be a rapid increase in the pulse rate due to quickened heart beat as result of direct action on the heart muscles. Had the autonomic nervous system been under control of the brain any increase in blood pressure would have initiated a train of events that would eventually result in dilatation (widening) of blood vessels, fall of blood pressure and reduction of pulse rate to normal. In dysreflexia this process does not occur and the person may experience an intense headache that is thumping in nature, severe sweating, red patches on the skin and, in extreme cases, convulsions.

One of the commonest causes of such an occurrence is over-filling or stretching of the bladder. Occasionally bowel dilatation due to severe loading may also be a factor. If the bladder is being drained by a catheter, either blocking of the catheter or allowing back pressure to build up by not emptying the collecting bag regularly may produce dilatation of the urinary bladder, thus initiating the train of events. Continued kinking of the catheter or the drainage system may also act in a similar manner. Stones that may develop in the bladder and extreme sensitivity of the urethra to the presence of a catheter may also tend to precipitate dysreflexia.

Catheterization should, therefore be done gently and by specially trained attendants who will use the correct technique. Many times it is has been found by the centre in Southport to be safer to have a relative who has been trained in such a technique than an unfamiliar community nurse. It is therefore essential that all involved in spinal injury care are aware of this strange phenomenon and ensure the person does not allow their bladder to become distended beyond a certain level.

Though a simple catheterization may be all that is necessary, the worrying problem is that many general practitioners, particularly emergency doctors during weekends or even hospital consultants, who are not specialists in care of spinal cord injuries, may be unaware of this rather unusual vulnerability in a person with high

---

AUTONOMIC DYSREFLEXIA / HYPERREFLEXIA

Untreated, the condition is life threatening and can result in convulsions, cerebral haemorrhage and death:

* Occurs in spinal cord lesions at and above T6.

* Occurs due to increased autonomic activity after stimulus (such as distended bowel or bladder).

* Signal from receptor travels up column until blocked at level of lesion.

* Local vasoconstriction responses are activated, and the person experiences intense headache due to a rapid rise in blood pressure.

* Parasympathetic response to try to stabilize blood pressure cannot travel down spinal cord past the level of lesion, and so blood pressure continues to rise.

Management:

* At first sign of symptoms (flushing, serious sweating above lesion level, nasal congestion, extreme head-ache) take immediate action to determine cause and remove stimulus (e.g. ensure bowel or bladder is fully evacuated).

* If in doubt, contact emergency services immediately. The person's treating spinal injuries centre will have provided an information leaflet on dysreflexia at discharge for this very occasion. Present this at casu-alty. Do not assume people will understand what the condition is!

* Sublingual Nifedipine can be used to lower blood pressure.

Figure 1.6: Diagnosis and treatment of autonomic dysreflexia (adapted from Tomlinson, 1999).

spinal cord injury. It is therefore essential to encourage the injured person to take responsibility for their own physical care as soon after trauma as possible and to seek appropriate and timely help if they suspect such a situation may indeed be developing.

Summary

Spinal cord injury, both intrinsically and in the case of each person, is a unique form of trauma; in no other area of injury or illness does there tend to remain, throughout the rest of life, complete cognitive control with the inability to control the body. Although injury most frequently occurs in younger men, essentially as a consequence of cultural and economic factors, trauma does not respect chronology. Similarly, from the perspective of rehabilitation, neurological level of spinal cord lesion can only ever serve as an indicator of post-injury function. Clinicians must therefore be skilled in the application of their abilities to the entire age range. Correlated with such a wide range of ages is the increasing life expectancy of those with spinal cord injury; with a small number of exceptions this may be considered comparable to that of those who are able bodied. Complications of spinal trauma present considerable hurdles which must be overcome if adjustment is to be effective and quality of life maintained. The need for awareness of the myriad causes of spinal cord injury and access to appropriate services and support has, therefore, never been greater.

Further Reading

Grundy, D. and Swain, A. (1993). *ABC of Spinal Cord Injury*, 2nd Ed. London: British Medical Journal.
Provides a good general introduction to altered physiology following spinal cord injury and acute management.

Mumenthaler, M. (1985). (translated by Appenzeller, O.) *Neurologic Differential Diagnosis*. New York: Thieme-Stratton.
Probably the clearest presentation of the alteration in physiology following all neurological injury but now only available in German. If possible, borrow from the British Library.

http://www.asia-spinalinjury.org.
An up-to-date web site with useful database access and links to other spinal injury related sites (see also Organizations, addresses and web pages, p. 151).

2

Explaining Prognosis to Patients and Relatives

How Does it Feel to be Told You Won't Walk Again?

Introduction

Popular newspapers frequently print appeals to help provide treatment for emotive cases usually involving last-chance attempts to save a child's life. These issues touch the sensibilities of almost everyone, with broadsheets often examining in some detail the moral and ethical issues associated with each case. Such expressions of humanitarianism or altruism may be seen as evidence of a developed culture and civilization and tend to be well supported as to some extent they are anonymous, do not specifically involve the contributor, and enable people to feel good about themselves.

Everyone will experience some degree of misfortune in their lives at some time, the commonest being the death of a close relative. It is often only at this point that people move beyond the ability to talk about loss in general terms and begin to examine the implications to themselves. It is rare to talk of personal loss and even less common to speak with another who has themselves experienced a loss. The ability to talk about loss is in itself a skill, a skill which with practice is likely to improve and enable the speaker to avoid tactless comments and all too frequent embarrassment.

This chapter is designed to introduce the reader to the difficult area of how and when to break news concerning the extent of a person's injuries. It draws heavily on the writer's own experiences and therefore presents a somewhat skewed information sample. No apology is made for this; as each person who experiences a spinal cord injury is unique, so is the provision of information concerning prognosis. To provide some balance the chapter also summarizes the views of other clinicians working in the areas of oncology and bereavement. The aim of the chapter is not only to provide some pointers to good clinical practice but also to encourage the reader to reflect on their perceptions of how it might feel to be the recipient of such information.

Should People be Told Bad News?

Considerable research has been undertaken, examining the issues pertinent in breaking news of imminent death to those with terminal illnesses. Research tends to indicate that those who would have the responsibility of breaking such news tend to consider the person should *not* be told; only 50 per cent would tell a businessman, less than 10 per cent would tell an elderly widower, and only 2 per cent would tell a 35 year old mother with young children. Indeed it tends to be the consensus of non-professionals that it would be better not to tell the patient. The picture changes dramatically when people are asked whether they would wish to know *themselves*. Then around 80–90 per cent of people say they, personally, would like to be told. It would appear that most people think they themselves would be better off knowing, but don't realize how many other people feel the same way.

Interestingly, a similar picture appears in studies of actual dying patients. Around 90 per cent of those who knew of their impending death believed it had been advantageous to know. A possible reason for the reluctance of people to tell someone that they are dying is that is spares the feelings of the living rather than helping the dying.

(Adapted from Owens and Naylor (1989)
Living while Dying).

There is considerable evidence from other areas of medicine, most notably in oncology, to indicate that patients feel dissatisfied with the information given to them by their doctors. In a randomized control trial of treatment for early breast cancer, 51 per cent felt the information concerning prognosis provided by their doctor was inadequate (Fallowfield *et al.*, 1986). Most commented that having heard the word 'cancer' stunned them to such an extent that they were unable to attend to the rest of the information provided. The study also indicated that where patients were better informed they were more satisfied generally with the care provided by their doctor and were more compliant in treatment.

Although most spinally injured patients report that they are indeed given their prognosis at some point during the early stages of rehabilitation, they also report considerable variability in what they consider to be the quality of the way in which the information was given. Since few people, including medical staff, receive much training or have much practice in breaking bad news, it should not be entirely surprising that when the need arises it is undertaken with little skill.

> *I knew the doctor was trying to tell me something. He just stood by the bed mumbling about things to do with my bowels and bladder and then said 'and you won't be able to walk'. He asked me whether I had any questions but I could tell he couldn't wait to get away.* (Female, 34, T2 complete paraplegia)

When Should Someone be Told the Extent of Their Injuries?

It is not possible to generalize either the extent or timing of the provision of prognostic information to either the relatives or the patient themselves, as the physiological changes which occur following trauma and psychological receptivity to such information tend to be individualistic. For example, while a complete level injury may have a more predictable prognosis, an incomplete lesion, or a central cord injury (often resulting in the ability to use the lower but not the upper limbs) has a less predictable course of recovery which may extend over a number of months.

Similar problems occur in the presentation of information to those below the age of consent. There is little published information concerning the differential recovery in children as opposed to adults, although it is the author's experience that children often produce recovery beyond that which might be anticipated from initial neurological examination. This may partly be a function of injury to a system which is still developing, but may also be due to the initial limitations of communication from children in expressing those areas of their body which they can or cannot feel or move. However, even in those cases of complete transection of the cord, parents are often reluctant to allow exploration of older children and adolescents' understanding of their injuries.

How Should Someone be Told Bad News?

One of the most important variables, therefore, in promoting adaptive change for both the person who experiences the trauma and their relatives is the availability of structured, systematic support and information. Formalization of when to provide either is inappropriate as such provision must take into account the needs of each individual. Indeed timing of information provision to the point which an individual has reached in deciding to change their health related behaviour has been shown to influence the degree of change achieved (Rollnick *et al.*, 1992). For example, in deciding the best time to give a prognosis, a variety of procedures are undertaken within spinal injuries centres. Discussion with patients who have been treated in a number of centres highlights three main approaches:

(a) All patients are told prognosis on the day of admission.

> *I remember arriving at the Centre and being wheeled down a long corridor. I thought, this is just like Emergency Ward 10 . . . It was all a bit unreal. Then I got wheeled into the treatment room and this doctor didn't say anything . . . just told me to move my arms and my legs . . . I remember then I couldn't move my legs. So as things went on I got chatting to the doctor and I said, 'so what's the score, doc?' and he said, without batting an eyelid that I'd broken such and such and that the injury would be permanent. He said a lot of stuff then but I can't honestly remember him telling me I wouldn't walk again, and that was that. It was only about three weeks later when I remembered saying to a nurse I was worried about why I couldn't pass water that she said that's because of your spinal cord injury and then went on to tell me the rest. I can honestly say it was like being hit by a brick . . . I had absolutely no idea.* (Male, 23, T12 complete paraplegia)

(b) No formal prognosis is provided; patients become aware themselves what they are able to do.

> *It's only now, when I think back, I get so angry. No one ever really told me about what was going on. Sure, I soon twigged that I'd broken my back, but the guy next to me went through the mill. It wasn't as if the staff didn't care, it was just that there was so much emphasis placed on giving us written information that they seemed to have lost that human touch.* (Male, 31, T2 incomplete paraplegia)

(c) Patients are told prognosis at a time which is specific to their individual needs.

> *I remember a lot of pain. It was like I just couldn't get comfortable and this guy keeps coming up to me checking how I'm feeling,*

going off talking to the nurses and getting things done for me. I remember we spoke about a lot of things – talking took my mind off the pain a lot but I don't remember much about what he said except something about the longer the lack of movement went on the less chance I would have about getting it back. That really scared me but I thought well at least I've got to wait and see and that was good. So then as the day went by I got to thinking that this was serious stuff and I started thinking what might happen if it didn't get better. I wouldn't dwell on it too long though . . . then I got back to being more positive again. But after a couple of days of thinking it through and chatting with the family I got to thinking, shit . . . this is it. After the doctors told me what was going on I got so upset, but then as we settled down it wasn't as if it had come out of the blue. I still hated being told the score though. (Male, 19, T4 complete paraplegia)

In order to reduce the risk of false negative outcomes, and out of courtesy to the patient and their family, option (c) is considered the most effective approach. It is the author's experience that on admission patients often are in a distressed state, understandably anxious, confused, overly optimistic or withdrawn. The purpose of the initial consultation should therefore be to assess the degree of understanding of the individual and to begin to gradually increase awareness. It is a source of considerable concern that referring hospitals on occasion give false hope to families.

We got the phone call from the hospital at exactly 7.25. I remember it clearly. They said Tim had a serious accident and would we come down straight away. We thought the worst . . . you know . . . we're going to lose him. I don't remember the journey, just that it seemed to take hours. We were met by the nurse at casualty and she put us in a room and went to get the doctor. All the time I kept thinking Oh god he's dead . . . Then the doctor comes in and he says he's serious but stable. My husband asked if he was going to live and the doctor said 'yes' and then he said we could go and speak to him as long as we didn't say too much. Well you can imagine the relief. We'd prayed all the way that he'd live . . . as long as that happened we didn't care what else he was like, you know, but when he said we could talk to him, and that they were going to transfer him to [spinal centre] to deal with his spinal injury it was great. (Parent of male, 17, C5 complete tetraplegia)

Even a busy casualty department is unlikely to see a large number of spinal cord injury cases and confusion between repair of bony injury and neurological injury often occurs either because the family fail to acknowledge the distinction, or the distinction is not clearly made. In both cases providing more accurate information to relatives on admission to the spinal injuries centre often results in some incredulity and disbelief, and indeed further upset which might have been avoided. Relatives, themselves in a state of shock, are often unable to differentiate the distinction between injuries to the spinal cord and injuries to the spine itself. Similarly relatives are frequently unable to assimilate large quantities of information, and for this reason statements should be kept concise and general themes explored rather than specifics associated with the resultant disability identified.

Pacing Information Giving

In an initial consultation it is often appropriate to impart only one or two pieces of information stressing, for example, the need to maintain as normal and open degree of communication as possible. Relatives assimilate information at individually specific rates and for this reason global decisions to tell every relative a detailed prognosis at the point of admission are often unhelpful.

For the patients themselves gradual provision of information will often be most appropriate with initial conversation referring solely, for example, to the observation that the longer a lack of sensation and movement lasts then the less likely the return of such abilities becomes. Close liaison must exist between the clinicians, relatives and intensive therapy unit (ITU) staff to ensure the provision of accurate feedback concerning the comments and requests for information which the patient may make. Towards the end of a 2–3 day period, with senior staff providing further pieces of information, it is usual for the patient to begin to ask indirect questions either of care staff or relatives concerning their future. It is at this point that the formal explanation of prognosis should be given, by the medical and psychological consultants, with a key member of nursing staff present. Consideration should be taken to ensure that relatives are available at this time, although they may not necessarily be party to the consultation, nor indeed be aware that it is occurring at that particular time. It is the author's experience that in the past, when relatives had been informed that a prognosis was to be given, this placed considerable strain on their communications with the injured person. Similarly, to involve relatives routinely in the process of giving prognosis places considerable pressure on them to conform to an expected mode of action, which they may be neither comfortable with nor able to tolerate.

The process should be followed up by further consultation on a regular basis until each family member is both aware of the nature of the trauma and has begun to make some progress towards tolerance of the new situation. Hogbin and Fallowfield (1989) reported a study in which patients with cancer attending a general surgical outpatient department to be told their prognosis were provided with a tape recording of the event to take home with them. Despite the harrowing nature of the information, the patients were extremely positive about the benefits of the approach, particularly in assisting them to tell their relatives the bad news. Indeed the production of written information for both relatives and patients that outlines the nature of the spinal trauma and what is likely to happen in the first few weeks of admission, and provides information on who staff are, where relatives may stay locally and how to contact various service and support agencies, has been shown to be of particular importance in reinforcing the nature of the spinal trauma and likely implications for the future.

Few people receive extensive training in how to give a prognosis, and it is easy to be critical of how someone else has undertaken the task. However, the fundamental issue should not be who to blame, rather how best to promote effective, efficient and compassionate prognosis giving. It is important to note the needs of staff themselves after having undertaken this process. For all those involved the giving of such information is an emotionally draining experience. It is common even for experienced staff to become upset, and considerable time must be set aside following the provision of a prognosis to address their needs, through individual consultation or further discussion within the group responsible for the information giving. In the light of the views of the recipients of prognostic information, it is considered that the process undertaken has some validity. It is common to discuss with each person, later in their rehabilitation, their view of the method of giving prognosis.

I suppose if I am being honest as soon as I hit the water, heard the crack, and couldn't move my legs that I knew I had done something pretty serious. You hope that things will get better but as time goes on and people give you little bits of information you think, well I suppose that's it. But it's one thing knowing yourself but another telling the wife and I needed time to get my head around that. (Male, 35, C6 complete tetraplegia)

Some Guidelines for Giving Bad News

The general principles governing the provision of any information given during this meeting, and which may be considered relevant to all staff/family interactions are:

(a) Prepare for the meeting; wherever possible place yourself in the position of the person receiving the information – what questions might you ask?

It is common for people receiving bad news to react in a number of different ways, such as taking the matter calmly, becoming upset, requesting further information or asking to be left alone or with relatives. Wherever possible discussion with others who know the person or senior colleagues may assist in providing some idea of how best the situation may be handled and received. When confronted with this task, rehearsing what is to be said either alone or with a colleague is often invaluable. Such role playing in itself is difficult and it may be tempting to avoid it; however if staff find it difficult to rehearse, how much more difficulty are they likely to find when actually confronted with the situation?

(b) Be objective in the information given; lengthy circuitous mono-logues only serve to confuse.

Clinicians talk about trauma on a daily basis. Patients have limited understanding of technical terminology and for this reason it is important to provide information at a level which is comprehensible to the recipient. To begin the process of giving prognosis by a lengthy discussion of the physiology of the spine should be viewed in most cases as indicative of inaccurate preparation!

(c) Demonstrate compassion; it is important for staff to be aware that the emotions aroused in such a situation will undoubtedly affect them as well as the individual concerned, and imparting a feeling of compassion or some limited awareness of the process that person is experiencing often promotes greater calm and acceptance.

(d) Leave some hope for improvement; even in high complete lesions, there are a considerable number of options available to the individual which may not be apparent to them at that particular time. Even in the case of an individual receiving continuous ventilation there is the possibility of implantation of electrodes to enable the person to spend at least some time independent of the ventilator (see Chapter 7).

On admission patients often are in a distressed state, understandably anxious, confused, overly optimistic or withdrawn. The purpose of initial intervention is therefore to assess the degree of understanding of the individual and to begin to gradually increase awareness.

Close liaison must exist between staff, relatives and patient to ensure the provision of accurate feedback concerning the comments and requests for information which the patient may make.

It is important to remember that telling patients bad news is not an isolated event. Having been told they will not walk again it is often difficult both to assimilate that piece of information and the subsequent comments on other alterations in physical function. Similarly, even when a patient's initial questions are exhausted, there will remain a need to regularly support and update the person on changes in condition as their situation alters. Patients may also state on occasions that they are not willing or able to receive certain aspects of information concerning their condition. Constant review of the individual's case enables such issues to be addressed at a later date as personal circumstances alter. Indeed in cases where a prognosis of incomplete trauma is explained, by the very nature of the condition, some improvements over time might be anticipated. This presents the individual with a further difficulty in beginning to adapt to their new circumstances; being aware of the incompleteness, despite all attempts to the contrary, often leads to the development of inappropriate expectation which requires careful, systematic and sympathetic management.

Provision of structured support and information to all concerned on the basis of individual need and progress enables the transition from initial trauma to beginning to rebuild family life to occur most effectively. However, even providing information in the constructive way outlined above does not mean people will therefore respond in the way the clinician may expect. Patients and relatives should be encouraged to express their feelings as much as they need to, both as a form of relieving the understandable pressures they feel, and as a central aid to maximizing communication.

Factors Complicating the Timing of Breaking Bad News

At the point of explaining prognosis patients are therefore at a considerable practical disadvantage; not only are they lying down but they are also essentially in receipt of information regarding which they have limited knowledge to enable them to ask appropriate questions. Earlier research by the present author has highlighted the effects of reduced sensory input immediately following trauma (Krishnan *et al.,* 1992). It has been a consistent observation by the staff that significant numbers of patients develop acute disturbances in behaviour during the acute stages of injury, and that these disturbances are usually preceded by an array of abnormalities in sensory perception: patients complain about non-existent noises; feelings that limbs were in various uncomfortable and painful positions; and a variety of distressing sensations, including strange and vivid visual experiences.

For individuals with a spinal cord injury, comparisons can be drawn between the loss of kinaesthetic and motor feedback and the imposed restrictions of limb movements and sensory input reported in experimental sensory deprivation studies (Zubek, 1969). Harris *et al.* (1973) first noted that the immobilization of spinal cord injured individuals could lead to 'sensory deprivation syndrome'. Similarly, Ohry *et al.* (1989) noted the possible implication of sensory deprivation in a case study of duplicate limb sensation which arose in a 64-year-old man with acute traumatic tetraplegia. It is the contention of the present author that by recognizing the primary role of acute and substantial reduction in sensory input in the genesis of behavioural disturbances, it is possible to pre-empt such a development in the majority of cases. The research of the centre indicates that those with restricted social support networks are more likely to experience such problems, and for this reason relatives are encouraged to organize a rota for visiting as soon as possible. This not only serves to provide a varied, meaningful form of social interaction, but also acts as a form of displacement activity, giving a particular relative a specific organizational task which serves to give the relative an immediate sense of worth and value to the patient at a time when they tend to feel particularly powerless.

It is considered that a number of spinal cord injured patients experience elements of perceptual deprivation, similar to those imposed in deprivation experiments. For example:

1. There is substantial reduction in the range of vision due to immobilization of the head in a neutral position with restrainers blocking off both the temporal fields. The field of vision is virtually confined to a narrow inverted cone, the base being the ceiling of the ward.
2. The restrainers and protective pads for the ears produce reduction in auditory input.
3. A certain amount of nasal congestion is part of the altered physiology of spinal shock which produces some reduction in olfactory stimulation.
4. For several days after the injury no food is given by mouth due to paralytic ileus, producing reduction in and disruption of gustatory stimulation.
5. Depending on the level of lesion, absence of tactile sensation and proprioception produces an intense and distressing sensation of 'incompleteness' of the body. As almost invariably there is no

concurrent head injury, full consciousness is maintained, compounding the distress and confusion.

Zubek (1969), in a review of the physiological and biochemical effects of deprivation, concluded that the most important variable is the level of motor activity. For someone with a spinal injury, their motor activity will be severely restricted, if not totally abolished, but stabilizes over time (Crossman, 1996).

It should also be remembered that expression of emotion is usually associated with changes in posture or position; when we cry we often cover our faces with our hands or turn away, both actions being impossible particularly for those with complete tetraplegia.

> *When you told me I was half expecting it because of what I'd picked up earlier. But it still came as a shock and I was trying so hard to hold back the tears* [Questioned why felt unable to express emotion] ... *Well it's just not what we do in our family, we tend to be quite private ... I think I've only cried in front of the wife once. Part of me wanted just to be on my own but I knew there was a lot you were trying to tell me. I've cried a lot since and I did cry when the wife came in ... I still feel funny doing it but I suppose it's just something we've got used to. I won't cry in front of the kids though.* (Male, 38, sensory incomplete paraplegia T7)

In certain instances there remains a desire not to accept the diagnosis. While this may often be therapeutic,

> *I hear what you are saying but I'm going to fight it. I can't accept that I won't walk ... I just need to get down to the gym and I'll show you ... I'm sorry, I just don't agree with you.* (Male, 44, incomplete C6 tetraplegia)

in other instances it may seriously restrict rehabilitation.

> *There's no reason for me to go down to rehab. I've told you I'm going to walk out of here. All my muscles need is time to mend – I'll stay in bed until something happens.* (Male, 52, incomplete C6 tetraplegia; view reinforced by partner)

The frequency of such reactions must in part be seen as a function of the effectiveness of the procedure of preparation for informing of prognosis. Indeed it has been the clinical experience of the author that such expression has become increasingly rare. Similar failures in acceptance by relatives are again rare. Where this does occur it usually involves members of the extended rather than immediate family and may be seen as a reflection of inadequate information provision or as a coping mechanism which allows those individuals to tolerate the trauma. Resolution in such cases requires consistent and continued regular therapeutic intervention (with extended family this is often less possible unless they regularly visit the patient); confrontation is usually less effective than initial acceptance of the individual's position and systematic cognitive restructuring through compromise.

The process described for information giving following spinal trauma holds well for conditions where the paralysis is due to congenital difficulties, disease or illness and is either static or gradually deteriorating. The principle of a client centred, needs led dialogue holds true in all cases. The unpredictability of the progression of some diseases simply makes the need for open access to services more acute. This is clearly evidenced in the case of Albert who experienced demyelination (compromise of the outer covering) of the spinal cord following a viral illness.

> *I'd felt a bit under the weather . . . a bit like 'flu really. Went to bed that night and remember feeling restless and hot and sweaty and about five o'clock woke up and tried to get out of bed but couldn't move. The rest you know, but it was just unreal. I went to* [neurosurgical centre] *where they eventually diagnosed a rare condition, but because it was so rare they couldn't tell me whether I might get better or stay the same. The not knowing remains the worst bit* [the patient remains paraplegic to date] *. . . sometimes I wake up and I've been dreaming I'm walking and then I get so down . . .* [Questioned regarding open contact with spinal centre] *. . . It does help knowing there's someone I can talk to . . . just knowing it's there usually means I don't need to use it.*
> (Male, 45, sensory incomplete paraplegia T8)

Information and Support for Relatives

Providing advice and support to families is similarly important from the outset of admission. Expectations following admission have been addressed earlier, but there remain the practical aspects of how to support the injured person, and indeed how to ensure their own survival.

> *She came in last night. We ended up having an almighty row over nothing . . . I suppose I'd been getting wound up all day and she was the one who got it.* [Questioned further concerning the

nature of the disagreement] *It was something and nothing really. When she came in she looked absolutely gorgeous . . . she'd had her hair done and wore a dress I liked but all I kept thinking was I wonder where she's off to next, and I felt bad thinking that way.* (Male, 34, T10 complete paraplegia).

Relatives frequently bear the brunt of patients' frustrations. Such frustrations are rarely taken out on staff either because the person fears for the consequences or because staff tend not to react in the same way as those to whom the person is close. Communication provides the key to prevention for the majority of disagreements, frustrations and unrealistic concerns. Establishing honest, open lines of communication from the point of injury sets a framework for all subsequent interaction and those with psychosocial rehabilitation needs have a responsibility for ensuring the prevention of as much confrontation as possible by the provision of structured support and information.

Provision of such a system enables the patient, either alone or through discussion with other family members, to decide on how to spread news of their condition more widely. While adult relatives share the loss experienced by the patient, there is often the desire to exclude younger family members. Patients frequently attempt to justify this exclusion by stressing the technical nature of the hospital surroundings:

I don't really think the children should come in yet. Besides chances are they would only pull on the lines and mess with the machines. (Female, 32, C7 complete tetraplegia)

In assimilating the extent of their disability patients also need to begin to examine how their injuries will affect their home life. As with the personal desire to know our own fate, it is often easier to stress practicalities rather than examine the emotional implications of exposure to children.

I can't face the kids yet. Just seeing Jamie will remind me of all the things we won't be able to do together. I know he's dying to come in and I'm desperate to see him, but it's something I have to plan. (Male, 28, T6 complete paraplegia)

The underlying fear for most patients would appear to be that of expressing emotion, of 'upsetting' the children. The issue of control is also frequently raised:

Hospitals are not private places and it is one thing to express emotion with families in private but another when someone else is ill in the next bed. (Male, 28, T6 complete paraplegia)

There remain a number of practical considerations for the patient to consider in deciding how and when to tell others the extent of their injuries. The majority of patients will live considerable distances from the spinal injuries centre, with relatives often living across the country. In most cases, after immediate family are informed, patients need to decide how and when they wish to inform others. As professionals find difficulty breaking such news, so are patients themselves likely to experience difficulties. Similarly friends and work colleagues are likely to react in many different ways:

I plucked up the courage to phone Brian, a friend from school who I had kept in contact with. I don't really know how I expected him to react. He was very quiet ... like he didn't know what to say. Phil, on the other hand, sort of took it in his stride saying that it wouldn't alter anything, we'd still be able to go to the pub and go fishing and stuff. I could tell they were both upset, they just both dealt with it in different ways. (Male, 37, T12 motor complete paraplegia)

Responses may not always be as positive. Other family members, in particular, often report their frustrations at having to explain to those in the local community with whom until the point of injury they had little communication.

I getting fed up of people asking me how he is. It's the same old comments ... 'Well never mind, dear. I knew someone who did such and such and they're walking now.' I want to get hold of them half the time and give them a good shake. Just for once I'd like someone to ask how I am. (Wife of male, 53, T8 complete paraplegia)

Summary

There remain considerable cultural and social difficulties associated with the expression of emotion. As with the provision of prognosis, exploration and resolution of emotion remains specific to the individual. During the provision of prognosis patients will often apologize for their emotional expression of upset or anger, and while hospitals as institutions tend to discourage emotional expression, the responsibility of clinicians must be to encourage such reactions in the event of a tragic alteration in circumstances. In terms of principle, those responsible for supporting such issues must take into account as many variables as possible which may enable the person to deal with such bad news in the way most appropriate to their needs. Preparation is once again essential; prior discussion with other close family members – reaction to significant events in the person's recent past; critical examination of the individual's response to information and situations since admission but prior to the provision of prognosis – and close liaison between the entire rehabilitation team is essential in this respect. Similarly, organization of environmental factors should enable the person to be afforded sufficient privacy and immediate access to other important family members to react in whatever way they wish. Enabling and supporting expression, making time for the person, exploring personal experiences of emotion and promoting the individual's control over future events all serve to create an atmosphere of mutual trust and a focus for progress for the newly traumatized patient.

Further Reading

Owens, R.G. and Naylor, F. (1989). *Living while Dying: What to Do and what to Say when You are, or Someone Close to You, is Dying*. Northants: Thorsens Publishers.
Excellent insight into how it feels to be given bad news concerning terminal cancer.

Davis, H. (1993). *Counselling Parents of Children with Chronic Illness or Disability*. Leicester: BPS Books (The British Psychological Society).
Detailed advice on supporting relatives of children with disabilities. Specific section on supporting relatives when giving bad news.

Fallowfield, L. (1990). *The Quality of Life: The Missing Measurement in Health Care*. London: Souvenir Press.
Excellent introduction to issues related to measurement of quality of life in a wide range of medical conditions including cancer, AIDS, and cardiovascular disease. Good list of valid and reliable psychometric measures.

3

Rehabilitation in a Hospital Setting

Introduction

Once the initial stage of informing of prognosis has been completed there tends to be a period of increasing stability, punctuated by crises often resulting from interpersonal and family difficulties prior to mobilization. Patients often report alterations in friendships as those who feel able to tolerate the disability remain close, while others start to lose contact.

> *Being told his prognosis was probably the worst time for all of us. We'd expected something like what was said but to actually hear it . . . well it nearly cracked me up I can tell you. Anyway, having been told we found it hard not to say anything to Tony. Once we knew he knew what was going on then it was like we all breathed a sigh of relief . . . we could start planning and getting on with things again. Most Mondays when we first arrived he would often be really horrible. It might sound hard but I often gave him as good back . . . I just thought, if we let him get away with it when there's no reason we're going to make it worse for all of us in the long run.* (Father of male, 18, C5 complete tetraplegia)

Although the experience of patients following spinal cord injury is usually associated with some degree of wheelchair dependence, for a number of cases the outcome will be more physiologically favourable. Approximately 15 per cent of patients admitted to specialist spinal injuries centres eventually walk. Their injuries are referred by outpatient or orthopaedic departments, commonly associated with fractures or dislocation of the vertebrae, when the potential for neurological loss is high. Similarly, patients may often be admitted where neurological loss has indeed occurred, but who fortunately experience recovery of the majority of function.

The extent and nature of damage to the spinal cord results in a wide range of neurological loss; those who experience no neurological loss and those whose injuries are such that they may walk normally but for whom their level of neurological loss is no less catastrophic also exhibit difficulties associated with adjustment. These may be divided into those with some generalized or local weakness or paraesthesia of limb function and those who experience damage to the sacral roots of the cord resulting in management difficulties of the bowel, bladder and sexual function.

The central purpose of this chapter is therefore to critically examine those variables associated with coping and adaptation strategies adopted by individuals and families following spinal cord injury and to highlight methods of intervention that have been found to be effective for patients, carers and staff during the immediate phase of treatment.

Cases Without Neurological Damage

A number of referrals are made to specialist spinal cord injury centres where the fractures to the vertebrae are considered unstable, and where there is the potential for damage to the spinal cord to occur. In many instances spinal instability will be remedied prior to transfer using a number of fixation techniques, but wherever possible referring hospitals are advised to avoid such procedures and other conservative management methods are recommended in order to effect rapid, safe transfer.

On admission to a specialist centre, a number of options for management become available, each of which has specific effects on the individual's ability to adjust to their new situation. Patients may either be left in bed with traction to promote appropriate realignment, possibly in conjunction with surgery to provide internal stability to the bones, or be fitted with an external fixation system (Halo vest) which allows for more rapid mobilization.

Conservative Management

For those who require long bed rest the problems of isolation and disorientation are similar to those experienced by all new injuries (see Chapter 2). Their moods fluctuate, their emotions are volatile and they require the same degree of support and guidance as those with neurological damage. However, the experience of perceptual deprivation is less common, possibly as a result of the greater awareness of body position through normal kinaesthetic input to the brain, and the realization that the period of confinement is essentially finite. What appears problematic for such cases is the notion of having escaped significant neurological injury.

> *All my friends kept coming in and saying I was so lucky that I'd done no damage and that I'd be up and about again soon. Inside I was getting so angry . . . I wanted to say 'well you put up with being in this &*%$ bed' . . . It was like I felt I wasn't allowed to get upset because I should be grateful.* (Male, 25, fractures to T10, 11 & L1, no neurological injury)

Patients in such cases, despite experiencing no neurological loss, have still suffered significant trauma and the emotional sequelae are comparable to spinal cord injuries. There appears to be the notion that the injuries are somehow less serious, but to the individual concerned they are probably the single most serious incident they have experienced in their lives. It is the notion of perception of severity and level of individual experience which cannot be stressed too highly. *Their* injuries to the bones of *their* spine are the most traumatic event *they* have ever experienced and should not be trivialized.

Having escaped potential losses presents further difficulties for patients on mobilization.

> *While I was in bed I got to know the men around me who had various sorts of spinal cord injuries. I felt awkward on occasions when they asked about my injuries and when I first got up I actually felt guilty that I was starting to walk again when I knew they wouldn't. When I went down to physio I started to feel a fraud . . . I was doing most things for myself within a fortnight and I know everyone feels great when they know they can go home, but for me it was I think an even greater relief because I could then start pushing myself a bit harder . . . I didn't want the friends I'd made to see me do that.* (Male, 31, burst fracture L5, no neurological injury)

Although the person may be considered to have 'escaped' physically from their trauma, at an emotional level the problems remain great, even following discharge:

> *Although I'd spoken to you* [psychologist] *before discharge I have to be honest and say most of it went in one ear and out the other. I was so looking forward to getting out that I hadn't given thought to how I would feel . . . we were both so grateful just to be able to carry on with our lives from where we left off. But as you know, six months down the line I was starting to get that bit more crabby with the wife and kids, I was finding I wanted to avoid*

going out with friends, I didn't want to drive – particularly down the road where I had the accident – and I was finding it increasingly harder to think about returning to work. It was like I'd rushed like mad to get through the physical bit of rehab but not given myself time for the mental bit to catch up. (Male 19, fracture C1, no neurological injury).

Patients commonly re-refer for psychological support 1–2 years after returning home, for many of the reasons highlighted in the comments above, and usually require five to ten sessions to resolve their presenting difficulties. Although patients and families are made aware of the importance of addressing their emotional needs from the point of injury, their immediate physical concerns commonly overshadow devoting time to such issues. Indeed, given the effectiveness of therapy post-discharge, simply indicating the possibility of difficulties and leaving it until the person feels they are in a situation that requires intervention may be all that is necessary for such cases prior to discharge.

Halo Traction

In a number of cases of cervical injuries the use of an external brace, which keeps the neck immobilized by placing the head within a rigid support, is appropriate. Such a system allows more rapid mobilization than would be the case with traditional traction systems that require the patient to lie in bed. While this reduces considerably the psychological effects of prolonged immobility, the procedure is not without some risk.

I was pleased when they said I wouldn't have to be in bed so long, but I wasn't really ready to face up to what I saw around me. I think I hadn't somehow been injured long enough to understand what had happened to me . . . looking round the ward for the first time was a bit of a shock, but worse was the way a lot of my friends, once they knew I was up and about, suddenly tailed off the amount of times they visited. Suddenly, there I was up and about, but not really knowing what to do next. (Female, 23, fracture C3,4, no neurological damage)

Patients following severe trauma and shock need time to assimilate themselves into their surroundings and gradually synthesize how they will respond to their new circumstances. Although Halo traction has provided a method by which rehabilitation may be progressed more rapidly, consideration must be given to ensuring that the patient's own adjustment is in synchrony with the process.

Cases with Specific Motor Weakness/Lack of Sensation

To see a person walk who had previously expected to be wheelchair dependent is a source of considerable satisfaction not only to the patient and their family, but also to the centre staff. Incomplete spinal lesions frequently result in gradual improvements in specific functions over a considerable period of time; far beyond the period which a person may reasonably require hospitalization. Knowing there is potential for further recovery is a source of considerable support to patients and their families, but can cause frustration and depression where the expectation for further recovery is unrealistic or where the time scale is considered too long.

> *It was not knowing how much I might get back and how long it would take that really started to crack me up. Some days I'd push myself so hard that the next few days I was washed out. The staff had explained about fatigue in my muscles and that I should progress slowly, but . . . well you don't do you . . . you just keep pushing but not really getting anywhere.* (Male, 27, T6 incomplete paraplegia)

In such cases, close management of progress is imperative, and the role of the entire clinical team is to balance the desire to improve with the need for caution and realism. Patients who eventually return home with the ability to walk, despite considerable difficulties, may also be disadvantaged financially; those who are able to walk some distance but who require wheelchairs for longer distances often receive lower rates of benefits. Similarly those with spinal cord injuries which affect the upper limbs but who are able to walk (e.g. central cord injuries) report considerable frustrations in daily life.

> *I was soon able to get down to the pub to meet with friends and walk in under my own steam, but it took the best part of 12 months before I could manage to lift a glass with both hands; the loss of sensation also meant that I often dropped cups and glasses which was OK at home but so embarrassing in public. People think that because you can walk you are all right.* (Male, 44, central cord syndrome, C6)

Perineal Paraplegia

In no other area of spinal cord injury is the notion of 'hidden' disability highlighted in the above statement more pronounced than for those whose spinal cord injury affects their ability to control their bowel, bladder and sexual functions alone.

I'm walking around so my friends think everything is back to normal. Things couldn't be further from the truth. Every morning I have to check that my bowels have not opened and if they have it's another change of clothes. I avoid going out because most places don't have toilets I can get to quickly in the event of an accident, and going to friends is out of the question. (Female, 24, cauda equina lesion)

I don't try to mix with women now. Once things started to get serious I found it hard explaining the problems I had getting erections so I find it simpler now just to avoid it all together. (Male, 28, L1 paraplegia)

Bladder management using the techniques outlined in Chapter 1 is normally effective in avoiding leakage, but bowel management remains a problem for a number of people. Although medication is prescribed to regulate timing of bowel opening, for a number of people this presents the greatest difficulty for them to overcome due to the fetor which accompanies the accident. With careful management the majority of people will develop a regime to effectively manage their bowels, but the stages towards such an outcome are often painful and embarrassing and require sensitive management.

Paraplegia and Tetraplegia

Whatever the cause of a severe and usually sudden paralysis, there remain difficulties for the individual both in coping with their loss and in coping in their interactions with other people. The use of simple analogy often helps relatives to understand the initial stages of the process of adjustment more easily. Such explanations use the theme of fluctuation around a central pathway, with adjustment over time analogous to return to the path.

It's a bit like when our son was young really. When he first went to nursery he wouldn't let go of my hand. By the end of the week I couldn't get him away. Now it's like [patient] *is trying things out . . . seeing which way to be fits for him. Sometimes he'll be really positive and other times I could kill him.* (Wife of male, 34, T8 complete paraplegia)

Such explanations serve not only to help each person cope with the frequent immediate fluctuations in mood state, but also to place subsequent, more isolated, incidents into context. Patient and relative reactions to trauma may therefore frequently be seen as normal reactions to their essentially abnormal circumstances. Changes in mood and behaviour should not be considered inappropriate and specific intervention for particular disorders will only be relevant if the difficulty interferes consistently with normal daily living. The art of therapeutic intervention is therefore in enabling the individual and their family to avoid as many of the potential difficulties as possible, reducing the impact of those which are not either avoided or avoidable, when necessary treating those which require specific intervention, and researching those whose contributory role remains less clear.

The hospital rehabilitation environment serves as a test bed, enabling patients and relatives to try out activities and coping styles and to compare their experiences with others. Despite the depth of experience within specialist centres it must always be remembered that those who have personal experience of the trauma or illness often have great insight into methods of improving service delivery.

I remember the physios trying for ages with me to get my bed to chair transfer sorted. I just couldn't seem to get it right. I mentioned this to John [earlier inpatient] and he said why not try such and such. We discussed it next time I was in the gym and after a few tries it worked out really well. (Male, 22, C6 complete tetraplegia)

While there are dangers inherent in newly injured patients comparing themselves directly with other patients with whom they share a similarity in gross level of disability, close matching of 'new' and 'old' injuries by skilled therapists at appropriate times to develop 'mentor schemes' has considerable benefits, often for both parties.

I'm really glad you asked me to see Ray. Looking at what he was doing I could see straight away where he was going wrong. I suppose I got a bit of a buzz out of it . . . it makes a change from usually being on the receiving end and I was glad to be able to give something back to the Centre. (Male, 35, T10 complete paraplegia)

The process holds well for all conditions where the trauma or illness is either static or gradually deteriorating. The principle of a client centred, needs led, dialogue holds true in all cases. The unpredictability of the progression of some neurological diseases simply makes the need for open access to services more acute. Newman *et al.* (1990)

note that different strategies may be adopted in coping with a specific trauma as opposed to the ongoing stress of a chronic illness. There remain difficulties for the individual both in coping with their loss and in coping in their interactions with other people. Patients who have undergone their rehabilitation following spinal trauma find leaving the centre, even for weekend leave, initially difficult:

> *It was like everyone was watching me, the chair stuck out like a sore thumb. Going to the pub was probably the worst bit because all my mates were looking down on me.* (Male, 19, C5 complete tetraplegia)

Similar issues apply for those interacting with the person with the disability. Robinson (1988) comments upon the emotions expressed by partners of those with MS.

> *She gets very depressed and talks about suicide. When she's down like that my life is hell. Fortunately she comes out of it just as quickly as she goes in.* (Husband of female, 32, MS restricted upper limb function)

Alterations in role responsibilities after spinal cord injury can also lead to difficulties.

> *It used to be me that did the decorating and gardening. Now we get another man in to do it and that makes me so angry. And again, the kids don't seem to come to me for help with the schoolwork, just the wife.* (Male, 34, T8 complete paraplegia)

Robinson similarly notes:

> *My husband found it demoralising and 'unmanly' to have me as the major wage-earner. He is frustrated because he cannot provide for me. He also believes that as a woman I cannot understand how he feels about this.*

Models of Adjustment

> *I'd only nipped out to post a letter. I suppose I wasn't thinking. I didn't see the lorry and the next thing I remember is waking up here. You never think it can happen to you.* (Male, 35, T4 motor complete paraplegia)

Those who are healthy take their health for granted. However, 14 per cent of all adults over 16 have one or more disabilities, and approximately 13 per cent of this number will have a primary neurological cause for their disability. A reasonable estimate is that a typical district in England (pop. 250,000) will contain 4–5,000 people over 16 with a disabling neurological disease of whom 1,500 will be so disabled as to require help for most of their daily activities (Wade and Langton-Hewer, 1987; Martin *et al.*, 1988). It does not just happen to other people.

Researchers have examined in detail those factors associated with adjustment to changes in physical circumstances. Early research (Weller and Miller, 1977) examined whether personality variables affected response to spinal trauma and while it may be concluded that premorbid behaviour must influence such responses, the causal relationship remains less clear. Peyser *et al.* (1980), for example, examined whether the euphoric state noted in patients with multiple sclerosis (MS) was part of the MS personality, concluding that

> It would be naive to expect all patients, regardless of their unique personal and symptom complex, [to] react in the same fashion and fit into a single pattern.
>
> (Peyser *et al.*, 1980: 437)

Similar attempts, in non-progressive neurotrauma, to examine specific personality variables as predictive indicators of response to trauma and the effects of personality on successful or unsuccessful adjustment have also produced inconclusive results (Weller and Miller, 1977; Ducharme and Freed, 1980). The major failings in such research tended to be a failure to address premorbid levels of adjustment, and the lack of standardization of the data sets. A number of other models of adjustment are based on interpretation of observational data. Shontz (1975) described a sequence of reactions people go through following trauma. The initial phase of shock, which may last a number of weeks, appears to be marked by three characteristics; feeling stunned or bewildered, engaging in automatic activity, and feeling detached. Second, Shontz describes an encounter reaction, where the individual experiences disorganized thoughts, grief, helplessness and despair, which because they are stressful often result in withdrawal and denial. It is from this latter stage of retreat that the individual begins to allow reality to gradually re-enter daily life and so begin to adapt to the experienced trauma. The model is comparable to the stage models of adjustment to bereavement proposed by Kubler-Ross (1969). Rigorous application of such models in the clinical situation can, however, lead to difficulties:

Member of staff to multidisciplinary team: How can you say the patient's ready to go home. I've seen no evidence of any denial or grief reactions yet.

Definitions of adjustment are open to interpretation. Many individuals with severe disability do not consider they will ever adjust, as adjustment implies acceptance; a situation many feel they never wish to achieve.

I really wish people would stop harassing me. I know I've got on well with my rehab but there are days when I just think 'stuff it'. It's like I'm not allowed to have off-days now for fear of someone coming up to me and saying 'oh it must be cos he's in the chair – let's go and cheer him up'. I get on with my life despite this thing [chair] *not because of it.* (Male, 19, C6 complete tetraplegia)

Use of the term 'tolerate' – getting on with life despite disability – is not simply a semantic nicety; it implies a different starting point for rehabilitation, one which does not depend on an individual having to 'accept' before they can make progress. Similar problems are associated with definitions of coping strategies which individuals may adopt. Newman *et al.* (1990), in reviewing patterns of coping in rheumatoid arthritis sufferers, cite two definitions:

- 'A psychological mechanism for managing external stress' (Lazarus and Folkman, 1984); and
- 'A mechanism which may be both action oriented and intrapsychic and is intended to avoid or mitigate the consequences of a stressor' (Cohen, 1987).

Others have attempted to examine why some people respond differently to being given negative information or experiencing a trauma. Crisis theory (Moos, 1982) aims to describe a number of factors which influence adjustment; illness-related factors, background and personal factors, and social environmental factors. If the equilibrium between these factors is broached, the individual fails to resolve any conflict.

When [doctor] *told me Jim wouldn't walk again, I listened but I didn't believe him. I know a boy who had the same sort of accident and he's walking now ... I still feel he'll be OK ... He's got to be ... he's all I've got.* (Wife of male, 40, T5 complete paraplegia)

It is certainly the case that elements of control appear important in establishing a method of coping with acquired disability. People who believe they have control over their successes and failures may be considered to have an *internal* locus of control; those whose lives are controlled by external factors and luck, *external* control (Phares, 1987). There is a second aspect of personal control (self-efficacy; Bandura, 1986) which relates to the beliefs a person holds that they can succeed at something if they wish. Estimates of success are made on the basis of prior observation of others and experience, and an individual decides whether to undertake an activity according to their expectation that the activity, if properly carried out, will lead to a good outcome, and that they can carry out the activity properly (Bandura *et al.*, 1985). In situations where people attempt to influence outcomes and repeatedly fail there may be a generalization from this specific area of no control to other aspects of the person's life. Seligman (1975) described this as learned helplessness and considered it a principal characteristic of those who present as suffering with depression. However, being exposed to repeated lack of control does not always lead to learned helplessness and depressed people frequently blame themselves for negative events which are beyond their control. The model was therefore adapted (Abramson *et al.*, 1978) to include the cognitive process of *attribution*. In this process people assess a difficult situation in three ways;

1. Is the inability to influence this due to me or things which are beyond my control? (internal or external control debate);
2. Is this situation long term or can I see an end to it? (stable–unstable debate);
3. *Is it just this thing I can't influence or is it everything in my life?* (global–specific debate).

Evidence from other areas of trauma and loss indicate patients' perceptions of the bases for control affect adjustment. Levenson (1973) developed a scale to measure an individual's perceptions of whether control over their life is self-determined (internal (I) locus of control (LoC)), or the result of external factors outside their control, such as control by powerful others (P) or belief in chance (C). Well-developed internal LoC has been shown to be associated with positive adjustment (Shadish *et al.*, 1981).

> You meet some right idiots and I've often felt like hitting them
> . . . they see the chair then you. I soon realized that it was no good
> moping around . . . If I wanted stuff I had to go and get it myself.
> I suppose it was just in me . . . in my family we all just get on
> . . . I suppose it comes down to how you're brought up in the end.
> (Male, 40, T5 complete paraplegia)

The inability of individuals to perceive internal determinants of control has essentially negative implications for developing psychological strategies to cope with their lack of mobility; those who see 'chance' or 'powerful others' as determining their development tend to be less directive or directable in therapy.

> *I can hear what you're saying but what chance have I got. No matter which way I turn it's as if there's always someone there saying here he is again, let's make it really crappy for him. Having the accident was bad enough ... then the girlfriend left, then I had the problems with the flat, then I get the UTI* [bladder infection], *now the sore ... I mean come on, you're trying to tell me that there* isn't *someone up there who's got it in for me?* (Male, 22, T4 sensory incomplete paraplegia)

Although stage models provide useful frameworks within which to view behaviour associated with trauma and disability they provide little guidance for individual intervention. It is also possible that the stages they describe are, in fact, partly the result of a long personal history of inadequate intervention and support, simply reflecting the current situation rather than how individuals might have adapted if their support and information networks had been more comprehensive. In the statement above, the person saw few causal links between the sequence of events culminating in the development of his pressure sore, and even less responsibility or control over the sequence. Numerous models exist which attempt to conceptualize the adaptation process through which individuals pass. Crisis theory exponents (Aguiler and Mesgick, 1978) contend that individuals maintain a state of homeostatic balance during their lifetime during which they learn adaptive coping techniques.

A crisis occurs, in this case following SCI, when the equilibrium is breached and the individual fails in resolving the conflict.

Attribution theory (Zuckerman, 1979) is concerned with the way individuals explain events, using certain degrees of bias in explaining their own and others' behaviours. There is a tendency for people to attribute positive events or success to their own efforts, while attributing negative events to those of other people. Attribution theory further predicts that the utilization of such explanations will therefore lead to different reactions to situations with different associated causalities. Three factors appear important in decision making within this framework: locus of control (LoC) (internal or external), stability and controllability. Thus if the cause of a person's lack of rehabilitation progress following spinal trauma is attributed to factors perceived to be within their own control, an observer would feel less compulsion to lend assistance. More help would be given where the dependency is attributed to factors such as a lack of ability on the part of the person (internal LoC but uncontrollable) than when it is attributed to lack of effort (internal LoC and controllable) (Weiner, 1979).

The search to examine the best processes by which adjustment may be made, the specific effects of traumas on selective groups of individuals, and the development of questionnaires and assessment devices which provide definitive scores by which individuals' progress might be measured, remain elusive goals. Indeed the very nature of spinal cord injury is such that no two injuries are ever likely to produce exactly the same level of trauma. While gross definitions such as complete C5 or T12 are possible, the net effects vary from individual to individual. Two complete C6 injury patients may both have the ability to push their wheelchairs, but one may experience hypersensitivity making the process painful and therefore worthy of avoidance; the other may have no available family support, be approaching retirement, or in receipt of compensation.

Clinicians have attempted to overcome this disparity to best effect by manipulating environments to maximize individual opportunity for rehabilitation. Inpatient involvement in the rehabilitation process has been noted (Norris Baker *et al.*, 1981) as predictive of medical and behavioural outcome; those who involve themselves actively in rehabilitation are more likely to be independent after discharge and have lower readmission rates. Although the causal link between individual circumstances and involvement is not established, the importance of clearly defined goals in the rehabilitation process is clear (Kennedy *et al.*, 1988; Kennedy *et al.*, 1991; Macleod and Macleod, 1996).

Providing goals and expectations for rehabilitation and adjustment is an essential part of any rehabilitation programme, but such programmes must also take into account the specific circumstances of the individual. While there are a number of models of adjustment which may be applied, in practice those which have most effect are all based on a synthesis of those physical, personal and situational variables that the individual brings to the rehabilitation process, the processes that the individual might reasonably be expected to achieve, and the net effect on the individual of engaging in such processes.

One framework within which such processes may be understood, monitored and modified is the application of functional analysis, a system which has been borrowed from the physical sciences where it has two precise referents. First, it is used to describe the nature of a mathematical relationship between determining variables and those which are determined; and second, it is used to specify the functional value of any variable within a biological system. While the language used to describe the process may differ depending on the theoretical or professional background of the individual concerned, the fundamental principles remain the same.

The essential characteristics of functional analysis in clinical psychology have been described elsewhere (Slade, 1982; Owens and Ashcroft, 1982) as has its application to specific populations (Jackson *et al.*, 1987; Glass, 1992b). Such an analysis requires

> the variables, for any particular behaviour or process, to be specified and an examination made of the relationship between those variables and the process. In this case defining adjustment, as the process, enables those variables which may influence its occurrence to be specified. Such *antecedents* may include individual motivation, family support, or the enthusiasm of the therapist (or community care team on discharge). Actively engaging in 'adjustment' (the *behaviour*) will therefore only become more likely if the *consequences* of engaging in such activities are reinforced. If reinforcement is not obtained, either from intrinsic and/or extrinsic sources, then the likelihood of its occurrence becomes less.
>
> Glass, 1994 p.56

Such a textbook definition overcomplicates the matter. It is more easily understood as the relationship between

$$A \longrightarrow B \longrightarrow C$$

'A', or antecedents, bring about a 'B' behaviour, the 'C' consequences of which make B more or less likely to occur again. For example, when we smile at someone ('B') we do so because we have learnt by previous association ('A') that we get something out of it we like ('C'). As the consequences are favourable (someone we like smiles back at us) the behaviour of our smiling is reinforced (made more likely to occur again).

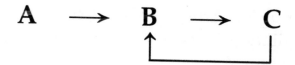

In some clinical situations, ignoring a specific behaviour which is inappropriate in the hope that it will go away (e.g. a frustrated patient may continually swear at family members who, because of their concerns, fail to admonish this when before the accident it would have been reprimanded) may only serve to exacerbate the problem; in other situations such action can lead to an adaptive alteration in behaviour.

Such interactions can theoretically be extended considerably to include not only interactions between an individual and their family and care staff, but also the involvement of wider public bodies and government agencies. A person, for example, who had previously managed to cope without assistance ('A') may be frustrated and become depressed ('B') through their failure to obtain benefit ('C'), which in turn reflects a prevailing political situation. However, limitations are placed on functional analysis to the point from which change might be realistically made.

It is possible, therefore, to design an algorithm to explain the factors of relevance in adaptation to spinal cord injury, on the basis of available research evidence (see Figure 3.1).

This idealized view of rehabilitation serves as a framework within which to view the potential for problems at any stage in the process. In this case an example is given (Figure 3.2) of how a pressure mark may arise. Whatever the condition or difficulty, the fundamental principle remains. Patients do not function in isolation and the role of family support and social structures significantly influences the likelihood of success of the rehabilitation process.

Other variables are then highlighted which may serve to hinder the process of further adjustment, but which in doing so also provide potential areas for intervention to improve the situation: in this case ensuring provision of comprehensive information and education prior to mobilization, organizing increased meaningful involvement by relatives, or providing psychological support to enable the individual to attain realistic expectations for progress.

Such an analysis may be applied at any part of the rehabilitation process outlined in Figure 3.1. The essential variables common to successful rehabilitation would therefore appear to depend to a signifi-cant degree on the quality of communication and information systems which operate. A detailed example of the utility of the functional analytic approach in clinical practice is included in Chapter 5.

Measuring the Effectiveness of the Rehabilitation Process

The process of rehabilitation following spinal trauma involves a wide range of professionals. Furthermore, their involvement should not be a sequential process, following on from intensive or acute care, rather a continual seamless process of rehabilitation commencing on the day of admission involving medical, nursing, clinical psychology, occupa-tional therapy, physiotherapy, and social work staff. Each has a specific role to play with both the patient and their family on admission and

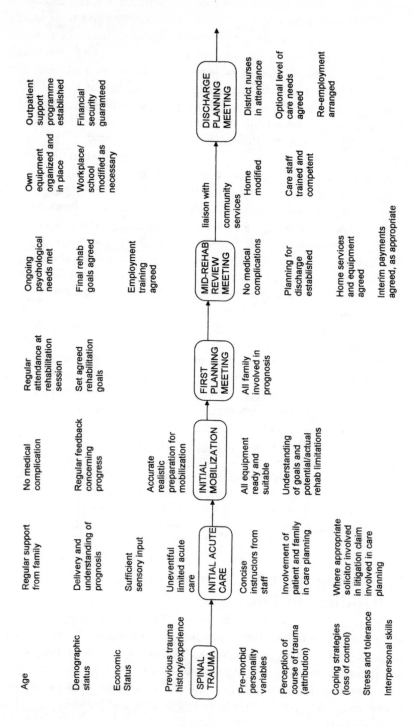

Figure 3.1: An idealized pathway for spinal cord rehabilitation.

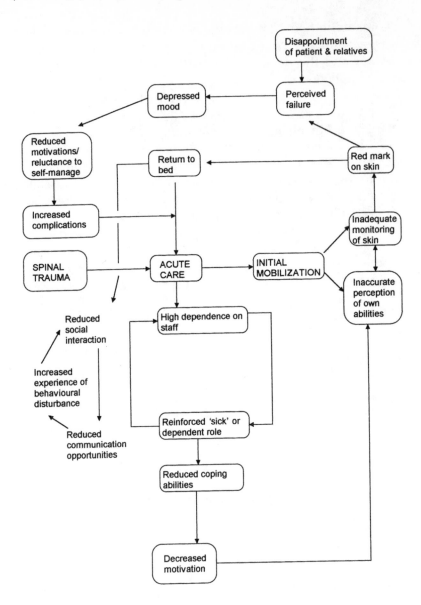

Figure 3.2: Functional analysis of pressure sore formation.

throughout the period of rehabilitation. Throughout all processes of rehabilitation, whether following spinal cord injury or any other condition, the central aim remains the gradual withdrawal of intervention, dependent upon assessed need, over time. Analysis of the processes underpinning rehabilitation has been the subject of considerable investigation in recent years. Whalley Hammel (1995) proposes a process of patient empowerment whereby

... rehabilitation staff become a resource, a partner and a learner, and the client becomes a problem solver, a goal definer and the person responsible for his own healthcare and management.

(Whalley Hammel, 1995:p29)

However, such a philosophy is not routinely applied (Glass *et al.*, 1991b). It is in the best interests of both the specialist centres and the patients who they rehabilitate, that the process of rehabilitation and return to the community be as smooth as possible. Rapid rehabilitation, on pragmatic grounds alone, is to be seen as desirable as it enables each centre to treat more patients. Furthermore, rapid rehabilitation may also be considered to promote patient independence, by reducing the risk of institutionalization which often occurs in long stay settings. However, speed does not necessarily equate with provision of comprehensive care and a balance must be made between these two variables to ensure that centres provide a high quality service which meets the needs of each individual patient.

The development of a reliable measure of rehabilitative efficacy has taxed leading researchers for over twenty years, with varying levels of success. Following spinal trauma there are a number of areas of mobility, personal care and hygiene which need to be relearnt, dependent upon the resultant level of disability. Assessment of an individual's level of independence with basic functions such as movement and toileting has been accomplished in rehabilitation medicine using standardized scales, such as the Barthel Index (BI) (Mahoney and Barthel, 1965) and the PULSES profile (Granger *et al.*, 1979).

The original BI contained 10 items each combining to form a maximum score of 100. Modifications to the standard scale have been attempted in specific fields of post-trauma care (Granger *et al.*, 1979) and in spinal cord injury (Yarkony *et al.*, 1987). Granger (1985) utilized a modified BI which included 15 self-care, sphincter control and mobility items, together with the 'PULSES profile' in four separate trauma groups (focal cerebral disorders, spinal cord disorders, other neurological disorders and lower limb amputees). The 'PULSES' acronym stands for Physical condition (health and illness status), Upper limb functions (self-care activities), Lower limb functions (mobility and transfers), Sensory components (sight, speech and hearing), Excretory functions (control of bowel and bladder), and Situational factors (psychological, emotional, cognitive, social and financial supports). Granger considered the modified BI *plus* the PULSES to be better able to discriminate between the abilities of less disabled individuals than the BI alone, and more sensitive to changes than the PULSES alone.

Yarkony *et al.* (1987) utilized the modified BI for spinal cord injury, which was altered further to allow individuals to score points when food, clothing or devices were provided and they could perform at least 50 per cent of specified tasks with them. Individuals therefore received some score when they required assistance for drinking, eating, bathing and grooming. This modified scale has been used to assess rehabilitation progress for a wide variety of lesion types, indicating significant improvement in self-care and mobility for those who engage in specific rehabilitation programmes. For example, the authors examined the effectiveness of rehabilitation programmes for those with C5 (Yarkony *et al.*, 1988a) and C6 tetraplegia (Yarkony *et al.*, 1988b) and noted average modified BI increases from 7.1 to 28.9 and 16.6 to 50.1, for C5 and C6 lesions respectively, between admission and discharge. Similar functional improvements are also noted in lower level injuries and which, in a three-year post-discharge longitudinal investigation (Yarkony *et al.*,1988c), continued to be maintained or improved upon.

One variable that might be considered important to the provision of specialist care following spinal trauma is increasing age. It could be hypothesized that functional improvement may be less marked as age increases and therefore the elderly are less deserving of specialist attention. It is reassuring to note that in an analysis of 708 patients aged from 6 to 88, analysis of the data showed no relationship between age and modified BI score on discharge (Yarkoney *et al.*, 1988d). Advancing age was associated with increased dependence in only a limited number of functional skills, and only for patients with complete paraplegia. Such results support the practice of providing comprehensive rehabilitation services to all patients following spinal cord injury, regardless of age.

The BI and its modifications have been found useful in clinical practice because the questions it asks are relevant for those with spinal cord injury, and it has been undertaken on a wide appropriate sample. However, the problem remains of our inability to equate what is a statistically significant functional improvement with clinical (real life) significant improvement once the individual returns home. The scale is further limited because of its failure to address communication and cognitive deficits. In particular the maximum score of 100 fails to provide a definitive indication of the individual's functional ability to live alone or their ability to engage in vocational activity. Probably the most fundamental difficulty with the scale is an absence of any estimation of psychological adaptation.

Functional ability in a hospital or rehabilitation setting may not equate with an ability to manage in the community. Indeed the incidence of marital difficulty (Crewe and Krause 1988), suicide (DeVivo *et al.*, 1991) and admission for avoidable post-treatment complications such as pressure sores (Mawson *et al.*, 1988) is testament to the fact that variables other than practical ability affect global adjustment to spinal cord injury.

> *I was a bit anxious when I left hospital ... everything was new and a bit scary. I feel I'd learnt to be independent but being back at home soon showed me otherwise. I got so frustrated not being able to get things off shelves, get into cupboards ... simple things like changing a lightbulb became big issues and I just got more and more fed up. It wasn't just in the house either. I'd expected some problems when I was outside, but it got to the point where every kerb and step was like a mountain and I even started to become paranoid like people were deliberately making it hard for me.* (Male, 32, T10 complete paraplegia)

In 1984 a national task force was established by the American Academy of Physical Medicine and Rehabilitation (AAPMR) and the American Congress of Rehabilitation Medicine (ACRM) to establish an instrument to build on the success of the Barthel Index by incorporating measures designed to assess other areas of functional activity. The scale developed is called the Functional Independence Measure (FIM) which incorporates items contained within the Barthel Index, but which also benefits from inclusion of further items that both increase the sensitivity of the scale and broaden its applicability to a wider range of rehabilitative conditions.

The FIM itself forms part of the Uniform Data System for Medical Rehabilitation which contains a minimum data set of diagnostic, demographic, functional and costing information. The information obtained through the FIM can be used to track rehabilitation progress from admission to discharge and through into follow-up. However, other authors have questioned the sensitivity of both FIM and the modified BI in addressing the attainable rehabilitation goals following spinal cord injury. Gresham *et al.* (1986) produced an index of quadriplegic function (QFI) which they considered best identified the abilities of this group of individuals. Recently, comparisons of this scale with the FIM have been undertaken, relating this in turn to upper extremity motor ability (Marino *et al.*, 1993). The authors discovered differing degrees of concordance between such motor ability and parts of both the FIM and QFI, concluding that the QFI, in relating more effectively to motor power measures than the FIM, has greater sensitivity and accuracy in assessing this group of patients.

There exist a number of measures to assess functional improvement following trauma, each of which has specific merits with specific populations. Attempts by the AAPMR and ACRM to develop a generic scale in the form of FIM to account for functional improvement in all cases of disability have so far met with limited success.

Relating Functional Improvement to Adjustment

Despite the availability and continued development of standard scales to assess functional improvement there remains a paucity of valid and reliable information concerning the importance of psychosocial variables in measuring and promoting rehabilitation efficacy. Granger *et al.* (1990) in a review of the reliability of functional assessment scales in assessing the impact of multiple sclerosis concluded that of the scales used, including the FIM, none were able to determine the individual's level of satisfaction with rehabilitation without the help of a further measure of affective state (the Brief Symptoms Inventory; Derogatis and Melisaratos, 1983). Even the inclusion of such a measure of individual estimation of adjustment fails to provide conclusive evidence of rehabilitative efficacy and adjustment as it does not take account of either premorbid adjustment, or the demand effects of the experimental situation.

> *I must have filled in a dozen or so questionnaires at various stages. I'm at the point now where half the time I fill in what I think they want.* (Male, 44, T3 complete paraplegia)

Quality of life may thus seen as the ultimate goal of rehabilitation. It clearly does not equate with functional loss as many people with quadriplegia report a good quality of life, while many lower level injuries report considerable dissatisfaction (Whiteneck, 1989). There remains the difficulty of equating functional loss (impairment or disability) with psychological adjustment. Whiteneck *et al.* (1992) attempted to resolve this by utilizing the Craig Handicap Assessment and Reporting Technique (CHART) in conjunction with the Index of Psychological Well Being (IPW) (Berkman, 1971) and the Life Satisfaction Index (LSI) (Neugarten *et al.*, 1961) to assess the effects of increasing age on adjustment to SCI. The CHART scale was developed to assess handicap based on the World Health Organization's (WHO) conceptual model (WHO, 1980) and collects objective data on physical independence, mobility, occupation, social integration and economic self-sufficiency, with high scores indicating low levels of handicap. While the scale provides an accurate measure of social role fulfilment from the perspective of non-disabled members of the community, it

does not measure the individual's own perceptions of their adjustment. It was for this reason that the IPW and LSI were utilized in their
investigations. The authors' initial findings indicate that there is a
slight increase in quality of life for several years after injury followed
by a slight decline over the latter period of ageing (Whiteneck *et al.*,
1992). There remains the challenge of finding effective strategies which
might overcome these negative effects as age increases post-trauma.

Other researchers have attempted to examine the longitudinal
process of adjustment to spinal cord injury and other disabilities by
including some measures of perceived quality of life (Krause and
Crewe, 1991; Crewe, 1991; Crewe and Krause, 1992; Ferrans and
Powers, 1992; Aaronson, 1988). Crewe and Krause (1992) surveyed
individuals with SCI in 1974, 1985 and 1989 using the Life Situation
Questionnaire (LSQ) which examined activity levels, frequency of
medical treatment, ratings of satisfaction with various areas of life,
and estimations of adjustment. The later surveys included most of the
surviving participants of the 1974 study together with a group of more
recent injuries. They grouped patients according to marital status and
found considerable differences in satisfaction with life ratings for the
married and single groups. There remain a number of methodological
difficulties both in the collection and interpretation of longitudinal
data and for this reason such studies are able only to provide overall
estimates of adjustment which lack individual specificity.

The increasing life span of the victims of trauma, the increasing
hospitalization costs and the spiralling costs of litigation and levels of
settlement make the provision of comprehensive and reliable information concerning progress and post-trauma adjustment all the more
important. This is true not only for rehabilitation in general, but more
specifically in the case of spinal and neurotrauma where the personal
and financial costs are most clearly demonstrable. Accurate estimation
of quality of life is therefore of particular importance not only in
planning and implementing therapeutic programmes, but also in cases
where litigation is possible.

*What do I think quality of life is? At the end of the day it's
knowing that I can go to sleep at night happy and with a clear
conscience. It's down to me feeling I've done all right by others
and that they've done all right by me ... not having to worry too
much about bills, knowing that with a bit of effort we can do the
things which as a family are important to us ... being able to sort
things out and talk issues through ... that's quality of life.*
(Male, 22, C5 complete tetraplegia)

Quality of life is generally described as a quantifiable estimation of
happiness or satisfaction with those aspects of life which are important to the specific individual (Aaronson, 1988; Ferrans, 1990; Ferrans

and Powers, 1986; 1992). Quality is seen as synonymous with satisfaction (Campbell, 1976; George and Bearon, 1980), and life satisfaction is considered to embody an assessment of life as a whole based on how well personal goals match with personal achievement (Campbell, 1976). Other components of quality of life include self-esteem (George and Bearon, 1980), health and functioning, and social and economic stability (Aaronson, 1988).

Problems of psychosocial adjustment are seen as the greatest area of concern by long term carers (Trieschmann, 1987) and are largely responsible for restricting return to work (Krause, 1990). Recent attempts to examine social adjustment and quality of life following trauma have lead to increased understanding of the variables pertinent to global adjustment (Krause, 1990; Ferrans and Powers, 1992). Jackson *et al.* (1992) utilized a modified Katz Social Adjustment Scale (Katz and Lyerley, 1962) with 463 relatives of survivors of head and spinal injury. Their results focused attention on a number of first order factors (relating to three main domains of adjustment; emotional/psychosocial adjustment, physical/intellectual adjustment, and psychiatric adjustment) which in turn highlighted a series of clinically relevant variables that corresponded more closely with those adjustment processes frequently identified in trauma populations (Glass *et al.*, 1997a). Ferrans and Powers (1992) developed a Quality of Life Index (QLI) which was used to assess 349 patients' perceptions of quality of life following renal failure. Their results indicated four major domains which were related to adjustment; health and functioning, socioeconomic, psychological/spiritual, and family.

It's all right asking me what I think is important now and how close I am to those things. The thing that still gets me is what I've personally lost: I can't run with the children, I can't walk along the beach with my wife. No one has ever asked me whether what I'm like now is anywhere near where I was before my accident. (Male, 37, C6 complete tetraplegia)

The most important variation from standard research into adjustment which Jackson *et al.* attempted was to assess the spinal cord injured person and their closest relatives' perceptions of their level of adjustment prior to the injury. Estimates of adjustment in the past have all failed to take account of premorbid function; the fact that an individual may adopt a more passive approach to rehabilitation may not be due to the specifics of the rehabilitation process itself, but simply be an extension of his or her 'normal' mode of pre-injury behaviour. Both studies conclude that adjustment, or quality of life, is multifaceted and that financial stability equates in general with higher quality of life estimations.

Indeed further analysis of the concordance of estimates of adjustment provided by both the injured person and their closest relative shows that in groups of patients at varying times post-injury (5 and 10 years) the major variable that appears to relate most closely to effective adjustment is the resolution of the issues surrounding compensation (Glass *et al.*, 1997b). Mean scale difference adjustment scores between pre-injury and present estimation of adjustment were greatest for those who either had or had not received compensation. Those who indicated significantly lower levels of adjustment were those who were actively involved in the compensation process.

> *When the people* [expert witnesses] *for the other side come along they soon see I'm not trying to pull a fast one. I can't walk and that's it as far as I'm concerned. You're made to feel like you're trying to con money off them, that it's not as bad as you're making out. I suppose for some people there will be an element of trying it on but most people would swap with them tomorrow if only they could walk again. I find the whole process a great weight around my neck. I'm restricted in what I can do because of the problems of adaptation and not having a car to get out with . . . I'm sure I could do a bit more for myself if I had some of the bits, but sometimes you think what's the point?* (Male, 21, T2 complete paraplegia)

Given the adversarial nature of the litigation process which operates in both the UK and USA such a finding might not be surprising; the more rapidly an individual adjusts and improves in functional ability, more often the lower the level of financial compensation awarded.

The Nature of Rehabilitation and Defining Adjustment

Rehabilitation programmes endeavour to provide each individual with the skills necessary to return to the community safely and with the ability to continue to move forward and progress. It is neither their remit nor within their abilities to teach an individual all they will need to know to enable them to cope on discharge.

> *I'd been home less than a week when I felt like getting on the phone and asking to come back. I'd had weekends at home and extended leave, but nothing really prepares you for what feels like the finality of discharge. I thought I knew it all when I left; it's*

only now I realize I knew so very little. (Male, 26, L2 complete paraplegia)

At the point of discharge following spinal trauma, the individual and those involved in their care and support should at least have a working knowledge of the physical effects of trauma, be safe and feel secure if in a wheelchair, and have developed some insight into the psychosocial effects of their trauma on all those involved in the process. However, these are what may be considered as minimum standards and centres differ in the extent to which other services are provided. Pachalski and Pachalska (1984) first examined the educational practices in an international sample and highlighted the needs expressed in each under general headings of physiological awareness and social understanding (e.g. the social and interactional skills necessary to maximize contacts among peers). More recently, in the United Kingdom, the Spinal Injuries Association (1992) produced a list of services which it considered spinal injuries centres should provide; few centres currently match these expectations.

Adaptation to spinal cord injury places considerable demands on the individual themselves, families, friends and care staff. Education of the family is therefore an essential part of rehabilitation which is often not addressed; indeed the support of the family is often the crucial factor associated with successful rehabilitation as partners, in particular, frequently become responsible for continuation of the injured person's rehabilitation involvement (Decker *et al.*, 1989). Social systems therefore play a central role in maximizing and maintaining the achievements made in the early stages of rehabilitation.

The role of each component of the rehabilitation services provided within specialist spinal injury settings is to enable such a process to occur. However, despite the best intentions of service providers, the reality of community reintegration is often less than optimal. In accepting the effects of environment on adjustment and the development of coping strategies, patients frequently have to learn to cope with considerable adversity.

I knew when I came home the situation would be less than ideal. Living in the front room, having to use the commode and not being able to get out all took their toll on me and the family. I'm not blaming social services, we're on the list for rehousing and they just don't have the houses or the money to do the adaptations I need. I just think, what a waste. I've had probably the best care I could have had in the world and for the sake of a few thousand pounds I'm not able to get on with life again. It's crazy when you think I've got a job to go to – I just can't get there. If they'd sort things out I'd not need to claim the benefits they currently give me. (Male, 28, T6 paraplegia)

Rehabilitation may therefore be considered an active learning process involving the acquisition, transformation and evaluation of new information in the light of the needs of the individual (Banja, 1990). An individual's failure to learn, and thereby tolerate disability, while in part a function of the individual is also part a measure of the effectiveness of the rehabilitation environment. Rehabilitation staff may find some difficulty in accepting their role in an individual's occasional failure to become motivated and learn new skills; critical self-examination should be viewed as a positive rather than a negative attribute. It would indeed be counter-intuitive if therapists assumed they did not influence behaviour as this would negate their entire purpose. Indeed the issue is not simply a function of patient–staff interactions, rather a reflection of the dependency culture which institutional settings often unwittingly promote. Oliver *et al.* (1988) indicated the influence of such a system operating at one spinal injuries centre where individuals described the rehabilitation system as 'engraved in tablets of stone'. For systems to promote an effective rehabilitation culture they must reduce enforced compliance with systems and structures and increase the emphasis on shared learning, empowerment, co-operation and support (Trieschmann, 1986). Indeed it is well reported in psychological literature that unless a person feels able to exert some control over the events in which they are involved, they will cease making the effort to do so (Seligman, 1975). This process, by which the patient learns to become helpless, often commences from the point of trauma and indeed earlier examples have been made available of the level of impotence and helplessness which relatives feel immediately after they are informed of the extent of the trauma their family member has experienced.

In certain cases, however, individual influences on learning become insignificant in the light of overwhelming social and personal circumstances. In these situations, the ability to take advantage of a rehabilitation opportunity is often similarly limited and for this reason the person may be described as either 'lacking in motivation', 'uncooperative' or 'untreatable'. The concept of learned helplessness is of particular importance in this respect as those with limited pre-morbid experience of control over personal circumstances may see little benefit from working towards rehabilitation goals, no matter how much a therapist attempts to involve the person in the process. Indeed staff, because of their own personal experience and training, may often apply inappropriate value judgements in developing rehabilitation goals, illustrated by the following two cases:

Paul had never worked before his accident, rarely rose before 12.00 noon, played computer games until early evening, drank with friends until the early hours of the morning and then repeated the process on a daily basis. We manage his bladder and bowels, make sure his clothes are pressed and keep him in pocket money. (Parent of male, 22, T8 paraplegia)

Brian didn't let the accident get him down. In fact he was back at work three weeks after he came home, organized all his own adaptations with friends and he and Susan are planning to marry next year. (Parent of male, 26, T10 paraplegia)

Asked which person had adjusted to their situation best, staff frequently choose the latter. However, given the conditional statement that Paul has severe learning difficulties then most staff review their opinion. In the light of their personal circumstances both may be considered to have adjusted appropriately. The question is not whether adjustment is considered appropriate by those external to the situation, but whether those whose lives are affected by the outcome are themselves accepting of the situation by choice.

Rehabilitation and the Legal Process

For a number of accident cases resulting in spinal cord injury, there is the associated complication of litigation, where negligence on the part of another individual may be pursued. In examining the medicolegal process, it is clear that the current adversarial nature of such cases does little to assist individuals to adapt to the modification in their life circumstances. Such a system serves only to reinforce disability rather than reinforce individuals' attempts to overcome their physical limitations. Those involved in litigation adjusted less quickly when compared with those who either had received or were ineligible for compensation (Glass *et al.*, 1997b). However there exist considerable opportunities within the present framework to improve this situation. There is considerable scope for a comprehensive reassessment of the rehabilitation services provided by acute spinal trauma units to involve well informed and specialist legal representatives within the care planning team from the point of admission. In those services which have developed case management systems, the central achievement of each service has been their success in improving communication between professionals. It is a logical extension of such a communication process that the interface between medicine and the law be formalized.

At the present time the Spinal Injuries Association, a registered charity established to promote and support those with spinal cord injuries, provides a list of solicitors to those who call requesting assistance. While such a system responds to the eventual needs of the individual prospective claimant there are often prolonged delays between appointment of counsel and first meeting. Developing a system of 'on site' solicitors as an integral part of the rehabilitation team makes for more speedy access and a greater understanding of the entire process of rehabilitation. Extending the role of the multidisciplinary team to include legal representatives should enable greater pressure to be exerted on those responsible for adaptation and community support. In order to ensure such an introduction is used to maximal effect it is essential that each team member has a clear role definition, and for this reason the appointment of a case manager is essential. Such a position may not, and indeed in many cases should not, be the medical clinician in charge of acute care; there remains an imbalance in perceived power between consultant staff and their patients and there is a danger that such patients may feel uncomfortable with the potential conflict which may arise during rehabilitation negotiation. Furthermore, while expert testimony is widely sought concerning the medical effects of spinal cord injury, there remains a failure to adequately address psychosocial, functional and nursing matters. As previously noted, comprehensive assessment of adjustment to trauma is a complex procedure which the provision of a medical report alone may not address.

Together with the emphasis on case management initiatives (see Chapter 6) there has been a growth in the number of facilities and private agencies providing comprehensive assessment services (Krishnan, 1994). The direct involvement of legal representation with such a team, from the point of trauma, can only improve both the speed and equatability of future settlements.

There remains a need to examine fully the nature of the litigation processes which operate in the UK. The adversarial process does little to increase independence, serving instead to reinforce dependence and disability. While the merits and pitfalls of no-fault compensation schemes are well known it is not the purpose of this chapter to question the relative merits of the system, rather to make it work most effectively for the client.

Further examination must therefore be made of establishing goal related financial recompense if poor adjustment (highlighted among those involved in the compensation process in the present investigation) is to be avoided in the future.

Summary

There exist a wide range of functional ability and social adjustment scales capable of measuring rehabilitation progress following spinal trauma. There is less agreement, however, over which methods have the greatest degree of validity and reliability in their application to spinal trauma groups. The process of adjustment involves a wide range of physical, social, psychological and economic variables and the relative importance of each will fluctuate as a consequence of the changing circumstances of every individual. Definition of those variables relevant to adjustment provides a framework within which the need for remedial clinical intervention and support may be targeted effectively. However, there remain limitations inherent in measures which take assessments of adjustment or ability at isolated points in time. For this reason a dynamic model to explain the adjustment process is essential.

Further Reading

Norris Baker, C., Stephens, M. and Rinalta, D. (1981). Patient behaviour as a predictor of outcome in spinal cord injury. *Archives of Physiological and Medical Research,* 62, 602–608.

Trieschmann, R. (1987). *Aging with a Disability.* New York: Demos.
Good overall investigation of issues and practicality of living with spinal cord injury in the community. Explores wide range of social care issues.

Whalley Hammel, K. (1995). *Spinal Cord Injury Rehabilitation.* London: Chapman and Hall.
Excellent introduction to the practical process of rehabilitation, through a process of patient empowerment.

4

Preparing to Return Home

Introduction

Returning home is the ultimate achievement of the entire process of rehabilitation; the fundamental aim, however, is not just going home but going home safely, with a sense of purpose, and being able to continue the process of re-establishing a lifestyle of quality through self-determination. The two factors which determine return home are:

1. Physical stability, in relation to the extent and density of the paralysis, with particular attention to mobility and bladder and bowel management.
2. The suitability of the accommodation and the individual's ability to be re-established in safety and with minimum amount of upheaval to the rest of the family.

However complex the process of making the patient stable prior to completion of rehabilitation, it is the accommodation that is available that will often determine the person's ability to return home safely. Rehabilitation in the *real* sense begins only after, not before, discharge from hospital.

> *It's only in looking back on my time in hospital that I see how difficult it was for me returning home. I had this tinted notion that I would just take up from where I left off, but even the simple, practical issue of bowel management, which in hospital I'd found so easy, in the home became a major organizational headache. I'd also half expected some of my old clients to have some problems taking me in my new situation, but never to the extent where some actually had moved their accounts to other firms.* (Male, 27, incomplete C6 tetraplegia)

It is the purpose of this chapter to begin to define those issues which constitute both the preparedness of the individual to return home, and how safety of the environment may be assessed.

Deciding a Time For Discharge

At a cultural level hospitals are essentially protected and artificial places meant for treating 'ill' people and the entire pattern of life inside is determined by illness. This must be contrasted with the rehabilitation of people with spinal cord injury who, once their physical systems become stable, are not ill but experience varying degrees of disability. It is therefore the ability of an individual to fully realize their potential on discharge that is the real measure of the effectiveness of rehabilitation.

The interaction between behavioural and environmental factors in promoting adjustment and tolerance of disability was addressed in Chapter 3, and considerable attention must therefore be given to the appropriateness of accommodation. *Ideal* accommodation is rarely available at the point of completion of rehabilitation and a compromise must usually be found between the ideal and that which is acceptable, given the fundamental need for reconstitution of the family at the earliest opportunity.

One of the first steps, after the implications of spinal cord damage have become reasonably clear, must be to discuss with the patient and immediate relatives the type of accommodation needed and how best to achieve these arrangements. Discussion of such an issue requires careful planning, timing and implementation:

> *I felt I'd just got used to the idea of the injury when all of a sudden I felt like they were getting me ready for discharge.* (Female, 34, T10 complete paraplegia)

Discussion with relatives from an early point after injury, and gradual introduction of themes to be addressed, make it more likely that the issues raised by the above patient can be avoided. Early discussion, however, is imperative if subsequent delay is to be made less likely; the rapid appointment of a community-based care manager with responsibility for negotiating social service and care input through liaison with a centre-based case manager is imperative.

Beginning the Process: Weekend Leave

This is probably the most important single event in the rehabilitation programme as it represents three major landmarks occurring together:

(a) It denotes that the person has progressed satisfactorily in their efforts to re-establish themselves and that they are safe enough not to require the constant vigilance of the care team.

(b) It is the point at which the individual may begin to realize the practical implications of their disability.

(c) It enables the person to examine the practicalities of mobility and how the layout of the house and local surroundings will affect their life in the wheelchair.

The first weekend at home, quite apart from the intense emotional experience it represents, provides a very practical exercise from which further detailed and complicated negotiations may be taken prior to discharge.

I'd waited so long to get home, but I never thought expectation could be so different to reality! The biggest shock was the nurses not arriving until 1.00pm to manage my bowels and then coming back at 7.30pm to get me back into bed. (Male, 33, sensory incomplete C6 tetraplegia)

The multi-professional meetings at this stage become, due to the available information regarding weekend leave, more realistic and relevant to the person's need. Discharge must not be decided purely on a 'medical' basis but as an overall consideration of the factors that determine re-establishment and reconstitution of the family.

It is essential to realize that for most people immediate return to their own or new home, fully adapted to their needs, as soon as their stay in hospital is no longer considered necessary, is extremely unlikely. Health and social care budgets are held under separate departments in most countries and the immediate availability of funding to undertake necessary work may either be considerably delayed or simply not available. It is often necessary for patients to alter their sleeping arrangements, by living entirely on the ground floor, and accept the disruption of family life as a consequence.

The alternatives are, unfortunately, very much less attractive and staying on in hospital when treatment has finished produces a series of disadvantages.

It all started to feel like a waste of time. I'd worked myself hard, the wife had gone through all the training with the nurses and I was itching to get out and get on. The week before I was supposed to go the social services came on to say the ramp they had said I could have wouldn't become available for another month and would I mind roughing it out. He'd never seen my house . . . It's got four steps at the front and I'm no mountain climber. That month was probably the hardest part. I was watching everyone else going to rehab and although the staff involved me in sessions as much as they could we all knew that it was a waste of time. I

> *started drinking a bit at night, got out of the routine of getting
> up, started dozing during the day, and then began to find it hard
> to sleep at night, period. If I hadn't got out I'd have cracked up.*
> (Male, 24, complete T8 paraplegia)

Patients begin to lose purpose, may feel they are beginning to 'go
backwards', and often find themselves becoming more and more
afraid to venture into the outside world. In the case of children, who
themselves may not realize the delay is occurring, parents often
become increasingly frustrated, and in extreme cases become angry
and project blame on to the hospital staff.

Specialist spinal units are rarely able to keep patients for extended
lengths of time as the need to admit newly injured people must take
precedence over holding on to people who have finished treatment.
Where operational policies of centres ensure prompt admission following trauma, patients in such situations accept that centres pay very
serious attention to the need for immediate admission, not only to
avoid complications but also for much better eventual outcome in
rehabilitation.

Therefore, although centres would not want to discharge a person to
a place where their safety cannot be reasonably assured, it is often
necessary to consider a residential or nursing home, or a unit for the
disabled, managed by a hospital or a local authority. Given the
limitations on global care provided in general acute hospitals, it is not
considered advisable to send patients back to the hospital they were
initially admitted from. In cases of particular delay, however, even
such an option may need to be explored.

The place where the person is discharged to, therefore, is decided
more by what is possible and best in the circumstances that prevail
rather than by what is 'ideal'. It is often hard to convince patients and
relatives that arrangements for discharge and continued support
afterwards are determined by trends in legislation that affect both the
NHS and local authority services. Centres have little power to
manipulate the system apart from clearly stating what the individuals'
needs are and making a strong recommendation that every effort
should be made to meet them.

Receiving Care at Home

It is important to recognize that the ability to maintain an adequate
standard of care at home requires the synthesis of a number of
components which are of equal importance to the physical parameters

of the accommodation. Apart from relatives there are mainly two groups of people who might be involved in care at home. These are:

1. *Community nurses* Support from community nurses is part of the statutory services to which patients are entitled under the National Health Service. Before discharge arrangements are finalized the community nurses attached to the family practitioner must be made familiar with all the specialized care that patients require. It is usual for these nurses to be invited to the spinal injuries unit and given some training and familiarization by the case manager, and to enable the patient to be introduced to them.

   Support by community nurses varies depending on the area in which the individual lives. Certain areas have better night services than others and the numbers of times they will attend also varies.

2. *Carers arranged by social services* During negotiations about discharge, the case manager in the centre would examine the possibility of having such carers as part of the care team. Again, this varies depending on the system followed by individual social services departments.

Both the systems negotiated through social services will depend on the current legislation that is in operation. In April 1993 'Care in the Community' became operational and this continues to make very radical changes to the system of care for disabled people at home.

What Makes Accommodation Suitable?

The criteria for ensuring the accommodation is suitable depends on the level of disability and the level of independence achieved. However there are consistent themes which are appropriate for all people in wheelchairs and these are given below.

Access

The gate and the drive or path to the front door must be manageable by the wheelchair user. Most entrances have steps in front and these represent the most common impediment. A side or back entrance may also have steps; and the entrance doors may be too narrow to let a wheelchair in.

Internal Structural Obstructions

The problem of room accessibility is not solved simply by being able to gain entry. Movement from room to room may not be possible because of narrow doors or lack of space for manoeuvring the wheelchair. The toilet and bath tend to be upstairs in most houses and the staircase represents the ultimate obstacle.

Overall available space

Space downstairs is usually fully committed to family accommodation and dining needs. A wheelchair needs a fair amount of space to turn around and generally manoeuvre. It is important to ensure that the use of a wheelchair in the home does not disrupt the living conditions of everyone in the household.

Maintaining Independence

It is not sufficient simply to be able to enter and move about a property. The person should be able to put into effect all that they have learned during rehabilitation to keep their dependence on others to a minimum. The layout of the house may prevent them from going into the kitchen and making a snack or a meal for themselves, and toilet and bathing facilities are often unusable due to the way they have been planned with only able bodied people in mind.

Retaining Quality of Life

Many aspects of care that are considered quite routine and acceptable in hospital may not be considered at all in that manner when the person returns home on a permanent basis. It is unacceptable to have intimate body functions performed by nurses, other attendants or by themselves in areas that are in common usage by the household.

It is a matter of much concern and anxiety that despite the excellent arrangements that exist to admit and treat people soon after the injury or illness that had resulted in trauma to the spinal cord, society does not appear to have a competent and reliable mechanism to provide for the logical extension of treatment and rehabilitation to the home environment.

Making Accommodation Suitable for Individual Needs

Prior to discharge, certain basic decisions must be made. The place where a person lives is not simply a matter of their accommodation. The locality within which a person is known, the social life they had established, the support from neighbours and the individual's general acceptance of the relevance to their life's needs are all particularly important. Depending on personal circumstance there are several options:

(a) A person may have been, at time of the accident or illness, living in a type of accommodation to which they may not have any difficulty whatsoever in returning; any necessary structural alteration may only be minor. Such a situation is unfortunately rare.
(b) Apart from ensuring access from outside only a moderate amount of alteration, such as installing a lift through the ground floor ceiling, or a stair lift, may be all that is necessary.
(c) Necessary alterations may be a major undertaking and involve building an extension. Whether the extension could be built into available ground space or upstairs will depend on various details, requiring advice from an architect with particular experience in housing for the disabled.
(d) Acquiring new appropriate accommodation would be the most acceptable move. This may be by adapting a bungalow or flat or indeed having specifically designed accommodation built.

Finance will naturally be the determining factor and much will depend on individual circumstance before the accident or illness. Whether the person had been living in their own home or council, housing association or rented accommodation will have much influence on the decisions to be made. Similarly, whether the person is entitled to any financial compensation in connection with the onset of their disability drastically affects the options that become available.

Care in a Person's Home

Being able to accept care into a home requires considerable accommodation both from those in receipt of care (Vasey, 1996) and those providing the service. The common complaint from families is the intrusion of care into their privacy

My home is never my own. I was so houseproud before Colin's accident but I find myself running around at all hours of the day keeping the place tidy because of what the carers might think. I know it's daft but I can't help it. The carers are so good and we feel so lucky to have ended up with such nice people, but I still wish they weren't here. (Wife of male, 46, C3 tetraplegia, ventilator dependent)

Addressing the issue of providing care is equally pertinent. For District Nurses and care staff in residential homes, there is essentially a safety valve provided by the number of people cared for; if a relationship is difficult there is at least the knowledge that once that person's needs have been addressed, they move on to the next case. Being a carer in the home essentially means being there and staying there for the duration of the shift and managing the situation accordingly.

Considerable efforts are made prior to discharge to prepare not only the patient and their family for returning home, but also to support care staff in their needs. This essentially centres on developing awareness in four areas:

- *Competence* Carers receive up to three days training at the centre to learn about the care and equipment needs of the person to whom they will be providing care. This allows them to practise learning skills in a supported environment, but also allows some relationship to develop between the care staff and the patient/family.
- *Confidence* As outlined in Chapter 1 there are a number of physical parameters which need to be addressed to ensure optimal safety for the patient at home. These are specific to spinal cord injured patients and care staff need to develop a working under-standing of each. Similarly, in the case of patients returning home, carers need to be aware of a number of issues regarding use of the ventilator. Allowing staff time to practise and share their experi-ences regarding equipment use allows them to develop a range of skills prior to providing care unsupervised at home.
- *Contract* There are dangers inherent in allowing the provision of care to be an all-consuming process. Over time carers will under-standably develop good rapport with patients and their families. Carers may, in some cases, be the only people with whom patients come into regular contact and although this often produces excellent working relationships, the boundaries between care and friendship need to be maintained for the safety of all concerned. This may sound dramatic, but there have been cases where carers have provided support outside contracted hours and accidents have occurred which could raise the question of personal liability. While it is accepted that care may sometimes be provided outside normal working hours this should only be arranged with the prior knowledge of the care manager or employer.
- *Communication* As with the issues of contract, maintaining clear lines of communication between the patient and the care team and within the care team is essential. Care staff are encouraged not only to communicate problems in care but also those issues which they as individuals have found improve the process of care. By

developing the strengths of each care team member, the team manager is able to manage the process of care to provide optimal support.

Care providers and patients are encouraged to contact the treating centre at any time following discharge for further advice and support. Such a process rarely develops dependency, rather it maintains an option for support in event of need; this is considered an essential component of ongoing management and avoidance of complication.

Recommencing Employment

One of the issues raised as a concern, in particular by those in work at the time of their injury, is the individual's potential to return to work. As well as conferring some degree of continuity and financial security, there are numerous psychological benefits to be gained from continuing in employment.

> *It* [work] *gives me a sense of purpose. If I wasn't working I could quite easily see myself slipping into the 'can't be bothered to get out of bed' routine. I come home in the evenings sometimes and think 'Why am I bothering' . . . but then I used to do that before my injury and . . . well I suppose I get a buzz out of it. I feel like I'm really defying the odds and doing something which is worthwhile not only to me but to the people I work with and for.*
> (Male, 38, L1 complete paraplegia)

Confinement to the wheelchair, weakness of hands (depending on the level of the damage to the cord) and the type of employment the person was in before the onset of spinal cord damage will often determine ability to return to work. It is important for all people to realize that with modern aids and environment control systems it is very rare indeed that an individual would not be able to enter into some form of employment, whatever their degree of disability may be. It is, however, equally important to realize that much depends on the climate of employment in the country.

There are a number of government schemes which are intended to actively encourage employers to take on people with disabilities. The employer may receive financial help towards the cost of necessary modifications to the workplace. The individuals themselves may also receive help by way of computer hardware and specific employment training to improve their prospects of continuing employment.

Introduction of computers as an integral part of the process of rehabilitation is an important step in the process towards re-establishing disabled people back into the community in a purposeful manner. Computer-based skills in data processing and design have opened new venues hitherto inaccessible following disability and various sophisticated devices using infra red, tongue and voice actuated controls have added a totally new dimension to rehabilitation engineering.

The Southport spinal unit and the local technical college had received a grant from the EEC Social Fund for their combined work to provide formal education and training in computer skills for people with paralysis due to spinal cord injury to allow them to proceed to qualifications from recognized educational institutions. This venture – 'The Southport Project '– which is the only one of its kind in the country has now been in operation since 1989 (Glass *et al.*, 1991a). Such a programme provides a model for a constructive and promising move towards definitive pre-employment training as part of the rehabilitation process which should be co-ordinated through each regional spinal injuries unit.

In the United Kingdom, social services have advisers with particular expertise in employment of disabled people. These people are called 'disablement resettlement officers' – DRO for short. The DRO and social services representatives visit spinal units at regular intervals and the unit social worker normally arranges a meeting while people are still inpatients. Eventually each case will be referred to the DRO of the person's own area but the preliminary work will be initiated during initial inpatient care. The social worker in each spinal unit usually has specialist knowledge as to how each individual should proceed towards acquiring detailed information and initiating moves for retraining or definitive employment.

It is, however, difficult for an individual to be sure when to embark on some form of employment. Much will depend on the satisfactory resolution of various problems of personal care, accommodation and domestic life, mobility and independence. Much also depends on the financial restrictions placed on people taking up paid employment while in transition from receipt of benefit.

I worked out that in order to make sure my family were no worse off if my benefits stopped, that I would have to earn somewhere about £18,000. While I think I'm worth that amount, it would take me a while to feel confident to get up to working a full time job and most employers would be understandably reluctant to take me on if they could get someone able bodied who they thought would be up to speed from day one. (Male 24, T4 complete paraplegia)

While the desire of the individual, the contribution of case management initiatives and the importance of comprehensive needs assessment in providing support to the individual to enable a seamless return to employment cannot be stressed too highly, the realism of the above comments cannot be ignored. For the majority of patients, returning to full-time employment remains an uphill task, and requires sensitive legislation if the situation is to be radically improved in the future.

For most people, therefore, coping with the transition into a new lifestyle following disability will be matched with the need to cope with the alteration from being a major income provider for the household, with often reported complications.

Benefits pay the main bills, but the bits for the children and holidays are out now. If it wasn't bad enough ending up in the chair I felt like I was being kicked while I was down when they pensioned me off. I know my wife didn't work before the accident, and she say's she doesn't mind now, and I know it sounds daft, but I feel I should be doing it . . . I've always done it. (Male, 32, C7 motor incomplete tetraplegia)

Returning to School/College

Adjustment to spinal cord injury in the younger age groups is no less complicated than for adult equivalents. The practicalities of return are frequently difficult due to the poor access arrangements for wheelchair users in most facilities. These problems are simply compounded in the event of a younger person returning to education who also requires ventilation.

Having experienced a lengthy period of hospitalization and rehabilitation, children require sensitive assessment and support to enable their return to full-time education, although parents frequently voice their concerns.

We had such a fight getting her back to school. Her sister was already there and she had been in attendance a couple of years before the accident. The major problem was getting a lift put in. The school applied for central money but found later that it had already been allocated, so we had to wait another 18 months. (Mother of girl, 12, C4 complete tetraplegia; non-ventilator dependent)

By the time the day came for her to go to school we were nervous wrecks. We felt that she'd been away so long, none of her friends would still be around and she wouldn't want to leave us. We were more upset than she was when we said goodbye . . . as soon as we arrived all her friends came around and were asking all the questions which as adults we are too polite to ask and she was basking in it! I had to remind her we were going and on the way home I cried all the way . . . but it was worth all the hassle. (Mother of girl, 9, C4 complete tetraplegia; ventilator dependent)

The return to school and college for those who require ventilatory support is more complex, essentially as a consequence of the need for management of the tracheostomy and ventilator, but is not insurmountable. Other educational options do exist either through personal home tutors which many local authorities are required to provide, or, for older students, through distance learning programmes such as those offered by the Open University. The central issue must remain the individual's desire and ability to cope with the pressures of education, and continuous access to specialist spinal injuries services remains essential at point of need. Well-established monitoring and community support programmes are available through a number of the regional spinal injuries centres throughout the United Kingdom, but such assistance for those requiring ventilatory support is currently available only through Southport.

Life in the Community

Having established a framework within which reintegration into the community may be provided, what remains to be explored is whether the system works.

The Good . . .

My care package provides for most of my practical needs. I wasn't married before the accident, but my parents and friends have remained a great source of support and through getting back to work I feel I have as much a purpose in life as I had before. Being injured has put into focus all those bits in life we normally take for granted; not that I would wish anyone in a chair. It's just that all the petty things I used to worry about no longer faze me. (Male, 19, C5 complete tetraplegia)

I've organized some private carers for the morning so I can get up in time to do a full day's work. It wasn't that the district nurses weren't helpful ... in fact they're great. It's just they couldn't guarantee to be here at 6.30 each morning so we all agreed the private option would be best. (Male, 23, C6 sensory incomplete tetraplegia)

I'm usually ready for about 8.30 and get to the office just before 9.00. I can transfer easily to and from the car and I find driving as much a pleasure as I did before my accident. Getting into the building is fine since the modifications and I have a toilet which I can manage to get in and out of. (Female, 26, T2 complete paraplegia)

Spare time? Not a lot but I enjoy socializing and playing basketball. Holidays tend to be abroad but I also enjoy travelling holidays around this country when the mood takes me. (Male, 36, T10 complete paraplegia)

The Bad ...

My pain is with me all the time although sometimes it's a bit better than others. The marks on my skin never seem to go and I feel like I'm glued to the bed. (Male, 29, T4 complete paraplegia)

District nurses come in twice a day ... my home help does the shopping. When I was getting up I had so many rows with them ... they couldn't guarantee when they'd arrive and it was often too late in the morning to get anything done outside the house, or they arrived too early in the evening when I wasn't ready to go back to bed. I suppose over the months I got rid of my friends; I only see my son at weekends but I'm getting to the point where I don't want him to see me like this. (Male, 34, C6 complete tetraplegia)

A wide range of individual, situational, financial and practical issues affect processes concerning adjustment. The issues raised in Chapter 3 show that reliably predicting who may and who may not 'adjust' is a more difficult proposition. From the 'consumer's' perspective the problem appears slightly clearer. With the benefit of hindsight numerous ex-patients reported cases where they knew another would either succeed or not. The comments most commonly raised include:

1. He always applied himself to the rehabilitation programme when he was an inpatient.
2. She was someone who you could always hold a good conversation with.

3. There were always a lot of visitors around the bed and when she first got up the family were all there willing her on.
4. I knew he'd be all right ... money was never a problem.

At such a global level it appears possible to attribute each of these statements with positive aspects of adjustment. However, some issues raised were more ambiguous:

5. He was one of the lads. Work hard play hard... always a good laugh and enjoyed his pop [beer].
6. I always found him a bit aloof; got on with everything though and was through the centre in almost record time.

Statements 1–4 may be attributed to 'good' adjustment but even in such circumstances they mask issues associated with the individuality of trauma and its resultant effects. Issues concerning younger age at injury, longer time since injury, positive employment status, and financial stability are known to influence positive adjustment (Whiteneck *et al.*, 1992) but the transition from hospital to home can on occasion produce insurmountable problems. Statements 5 and 6 followed a discussion with a close friend of a young man who committed suicide following discharge. Although both statements may be attributed to positive aspects of adjustment (dedication, sociability, etc.), in this context they would appear either to have masked an inability to accept or tolerate the disability, or an individual who had indeed 'accepted' his disability but made a rational judgement that life with a disability was not 'acceptable' to him.

Depression: A Word of Caution

There is a perception within the spinal cord injury field that depression following injury is universal. Indeed some researchers have argued that if depression does not follow on after injury then the person is using denial to minimize the level of functional loss (Burke and Murray, 1975). However, researchers have begun to question the validity of such global representation (Cushman and Dijkers, 1990; Elliott and Frank, 1996). Elliott and Frank (1996) criticise the methodology of available research for unclear and inconsistent application of diagnostic criteria, poor definition and measurement of depression, poorly defined and testable theoretical approaches regarding depression after spinal cord injury, little integration of models of depression outside spinal cord injury and lack of longitudinal study.

As clinicians view each case with spinal cord injury individually, so they must assess the likelihood and implications of depression.

Suicide

The factors associated with suicide have been a source of considerable research investigation for a number of years (Hawton, 1987). Early writers attempted to produce a clear distinction between attempted and completed suicide, although more recent research has argued such a distinction to be less warranted (MacLeod *et al.*, 1992). Rates of suicide attempts and completed episodes for both sexes show an increase with age, social class, and environmental variables (Office of Health Economics, 1981). Among the spinal injured population there has been little objective examination of the factors associated with suicidal behaviour, with most studies concentrating on incidence (Nyquist and Bors, 1967; Judd and Brown, 1992). In this respect suicide following spinal cord injury is reported to be significantly higher among the spinal cord injured population, accounting for between 4–21 per cent of all deaths. DeVivo *et al.* (1991) reported suicide to be one of the main causes of death in cases of traumatic paraplegia, the main cause of death among those with complete paraplegia and the second highest cause of death for those with incomplete paraplegia. The same trend was not found among those with tetraplegia. Within this latter group the desire to end life may be high, but the ability or opportunity is low; or the higher levels of attendant care need provide a 'safety barrier' to reduce suicidal thought; it is certainly the case that those who are ventilator dependent view the support of close family as a key coping mechanism (see Chapter 6).

What remains clear from most research is the frequency with which people experience significant life events in the months preceding the attempt, and the greater the significance they attach to them (Paykel *et al.*, 1975), the increased likelihood of their having experienced early loss, death or other traumas within the family (Maris, 1981). More recent links with perceived hopelessness have also been examined (Beck *et al.*, 1974).

The problem of prevention of primary and secondary attempts remains. Hirsch *et al.* (1982) note that the impulsivity of suicide and the fact that it is a 'multifaceted state defined by its outcome' make the task of lessening risk and repetition a difficult one. The task is further complicated by personality predisposition, affective state and social factors all of which interact and none of which can be said to predominate. Perhaps the greatest challenge for rehabilitation professionals faced with an 'incomplete' suicide case is to develop a meaningful structure within which social and intrapersonal skills may be developed to provide some meaning for continued life.

Summary

Following the occurrence of spinal cord injury, families undergo a radical transformation of lifestyle and reappraisal of future need. Clinicians must be aware of, and apply, reliable and objective measures of diagnosis for depression and suicidal ideation and examine expressions of affective distress individually; there remains a perception of stigma associated with being 'labelled' as experiencing distress. Such correctness should not be at the expense of those who are clearly in distress, and if the desperation which frequently results in severe depression and suicide is to be reduced, what appears more relevant for future research is the need to concentrate on the cognitions and social processes which enable people to cope with significant stressors in their lives.

The transition from the inpatient phase of rehabilitation to social reintegration is best achieved gradually. However, the move from hospital to community reflects the operation of two distinct processes and it is clear from other research (Marincek, 1988) that where process boundaries are crossed responsibilities become less clear. It is uncommon for living accommodation to be suitably adapted at the completion of rehabilitation, and it is rarely considered appropriate at that point for the injured person to return to the referring hospital as the likelihood of complications developing is high. Therefore patients and their families frequently have to cope in less than ideal environmental and personal circumstances for considerable periods of time before some improvement in quality may be effected. This is rarely due to inefficiencies of effort on the part of hospital and community staff, but represents more a general crisis in funding. It appears an iniquity that means tested funding of modification costs should only take into account income and not expenditure. The numerous examples of families who were barely managing to survive financially before disability, being placed in financial turmoil at a time of considerable desperation by the occurrence of disability, require attention and modification to existing legislation.

Further Reading

Vasey, S. (1996). The experience of care. In G. Hales (Ed.) *Beyond Disability: Towards an Enabling Society*. London: Sage Publications, pp. 82–87.
Excellent personal account of the positive and negative effects of having carers in your own home.

Whiteneck, G.G., Charlifue, S.W., Gerhart, K. *et al.* (Eds) (1993). *Aging with Spinal Cord Injury*. New York: Demos.
Most comprehensive source of information concerning long-term effects and implications of spinal cord injury. Clearly written chapters covering all aspects of the ageing process: physical, social and psychological issues.

Hunter, J. (1988). *Bridging the Gap: Case Management and Advocacy for People with Physical Disabilities*. London: King Edward's Fund for London.
Good introduction to the need for comprehensive planning and support in the community. Makes excellent suggestions regarding service planning and legislative issues.

Elliott, T.R. and Frank, R.G. (1996). Depression following spinal cord injury. *Archives of Physical Medicine and Rehabilitation, 77*, 816–823.
Critical review of current status of understanding of depression and application of appropriate methodology for future research.

DeVivo, M.J., Black, K.J., Richards, J.S. and Stover, S.L. (1991). Suicide following spinal cord injury. Paraplegia, 29, 9, 620–627.
Comprehensive review of available literature and suggestions for future research.

5

Sexuality and Sexual Functioning

Introduction

In view of the wide age range at which people experience spinal trauma, there will be those who were sexually experienced before their trauma and those who were not. Whether the individual is first beginning to experience the desire to explore sexual issues or requires information or advice concerning their altered situation, the fundamental basis to discussion remains the same: each individual's sexuality remains a unique expression of who they are and support services must therefore be sensitive to individual need.

> *I just got the feeling that* [the nurse] *didn't feel comfortable with the issue. It's not something I can really put into words . . . she was very nice about it . . . I just felt I really wish I hadn't started this.* (Female, 37, C6 motor complete tetraplegia)

It is important not to view sexual behaviour in isolation, as intercourse for most couples, irrespective of physical ability, tends to arise as an expression of the overall quality of their relationship.

Sex, along with death, remains a taboo topic despite the increasing exploration of sexual issues in the entire range of available media. Exploration of this topic is not, therefore, something with which all clinical staff will feel comfortable and this is to be expected. The purpose of this chapter is to provide an information framework from which those who do wish to explore the issue in more depth may make further inquiry.

Sexual Behaviour and Adjustment

Investigators have attempted to evaluate individual factors associated with overall quality of interpersonal relationships by assessment of

94

issues such as self-concept (Nagler, 1950), and body image (Ryan, 1961). Indeed the whole area of adjustment to disability is essentially a 'longitudinal multifaceted concept'; changes occur throughout life which are influenced not only by functional independence, but also social, psychological, economic and political variables (Whiteneck *et al.*, 1992). Seen in this context sexuality is therefore a dynamic concept itself, being a variable which, dependent on experience prior to trauma, both influences and is influenced by the factors associated with trauma and disability.

> *If you'd told me before the accident in 12 months I'd be having* [sexual] *problems, I'd have laughed at you. Our love making was brilliant, and even while I was in hospital I really fancied sex. It was just when we got home, the catheter kept leaking, getting round the house was a pain, I couldn't get out easily, he was tired, I was tired, I felt like I was just a spare part . . . I could tell things weren't right but there never seemed the right time to talk about it . . . I didn't want to put on him any more than I was doing.* (Female 43, T8 complete paraplegia)

While the majority of people with neurological disease and trauma will have a primary organic cause for their erectile and ejaculatory disorders or ablated vaginal sensation, there are often considerable degrees of psychological overlay which reduce both the frequency and enjoyment of sexual activity.

Partners may feel reluctant or unable to engage in sexual activity due to over-emphasis on their caring role – changing from nurse to lover is a difficult cognitive transformation; and those whose trauma is incomplete may experience performance anxieties during preparation for discharge which are exacerbated on return to the family home.

> [Discussion following first weekend leave] *I suppose I built it up too much. We were home for around 8.00 and by the time we'd eaten and got rid of all the visitors . . . they meant well but looking back I think it was too much . . . and by the time we'd sorted me out I couldn't have raised a smile . . . but you feel this pressure . . . it must be something to do with being a man . . . the wife was fine about it but I just felt a bloody fool.* (Male, 32, L2 incomplete paraplegia; sensory loss)

Similarly, for women, the common failures of rehabilitation centres to discuss sexuality and body image often produce difficulties beyond the influence of purely physical factors (Harrison *et al.*, 1995). It had been the experience of the author, in counselling young adults with spina bifida, that sexual awareness is often poorly developed, which often reflects the unwitting desire of families and the community to treat the individual as though still a child, and the failure of child services to address such individuals' normal adolescent sexual developmental needs.

Sexual Function

A wide variety of texts exist which deal in detail with the physiological effects of spinal cord injury on erectile function, vaginal sensitivity, ejaculatory and orgasmic capability and conception. Sexual function and arousal in both men and women occur in response to either stimulation (reflexogenic) or desire (psychogenic). Those with spinal cord injury require comprehensive assessment of the level and degree of cord damage (to assess the effects on sexual function), followed by assessment of the degree of damage to upper and lower motor neurones (by testing bulbocavernosal and anal wink reflexes). In neurological terms male erection is comparable to female lubrication, and male ejaculation comparable to contraction of the pelvic floor, perineum and anal sphincter.

It is considered important in the context of this chapter to dispel some commonly held misconceptions regarding sexual function:

- Women with spinal cord injuries may still experience orgasm after injury.
- Most men can still achieve erection using various methods including intercavernous injection of vasodilatory medications.
- Men with low level injuries are more likely to experience unassisted ejaculation, but less likely to experience spontaneous erection; the converse exists for men with higher level spinal cord injuries.
- Men with spinal cord injuries often remain able to father children either through normal ejaculatory processes or with vibratory or electroejaculatory assistance.
- Women with spinal cord injury are rarely impaired in their ability to conceive and tolerate pregnancy, and the majority may experience vaginal delivery.

There remains sexual life after spinal cord injury!

I suppose I was fortunate, yes. Bill and I had always been open in discussing what we liked during sex. After the accident we read a few books to pass time in hospital and I developed the idea that orgasm for me was out. It would be an understatement to say I was pleased to prove that one wrong. Bill only has to stroke my neck in a certain way and I get such a feeling . . . (Female, 52, C7 complete tetraplegia)

Following return home and a reasonable settling in period, couples have had the opportunity to experiment and find out what can and cannot be achieved. The provision of appropriate counselling and information prior to discharge is therefore imperative in order that expectations may be matched with the individual's physical capabilities. Part of this process involves explanation of the effects of altered physiology and the treatment methods available.

Orgasm

Women widely report the experience of orgasm which feels to them as good as before injury, even though it may not be the same. The physiological evidence in support of women's reported experience is limited. Internal changes do still occur during sexual activity following injury, such as increase in heart rate and perspiration, and willingness to experiment and establish new erogenous areas not affected by the trauma undoubtedly leads to greater communication between partners and a desire to focus on new experiences. Whether women are experiencing recollection of earlier orgasmic experience or 'true' orgasm remains open to further debate. Perry and Whipple (1981) identified the hypogastric plexus and pelvic nerve as the sensory pathways in sexual response where vaginal stimulation occurs. Komisaruk and Whipple (1994) have hypothesized an additional pathway, the vagus nerve (which directly links the cervix and brain and bypasses the spinal cord), as a reason why women often retain orgasmic ability after spinal cord injury. Evidence from some women who were not sexually active before their accident and others who were anorgasmic in their relationships would suggest that they too experience pleasure comparable with what they consider to be orgasm. Taking each factor into account, personal experiences of pleasure remain simply that:

I honestly don't care what the textbooks say . . . I know what I feel and that's good enough for me. (Female, 22, C4 complete tetraplegia, non-ventilated)

Penile Erection

The experience of erection in men is similarly linked with personal desire. In the majority of cases the ability to experience psychogenic erections, when seeing or being involved in situations which before the accident would produce erections, is usually ablated. Similarly the experience of reflex erection, during physical stimulation of the penis, is frequently spared although the reliability of maintaining tumescence by such a method during times of sexual activity is less predictable and often leads to frustration for both partners.

Erections normally occur in response to sexual stimulation which, via the hypogastric and pelvic nerves, promotes the release of nitric oxide (NO) from neurons of the corpus cavernosum and initiates a string of chemical processes which result in erection (see Figure 5.1 below).

NO activates guanylate cyclase, allowing production of cyclic guanosine monophosphate (cGMP) which causes smooth muscle relaxation. As the muscles of the corpus cavernosum relax, corporal sacs fill with blood which, in turn, increases the pressure on the veins. This allows blood to leave the sacs, increases intercavernosal pressure and results in the penis becoming erect.

The thoracolumbar and sacral cord have specific roles in mediating erection and are often disrupted following spinal cord injury.

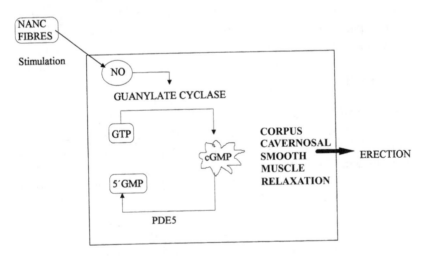

KEY

cGMP	=	cyclic guanosine monophosphate
5'GMp	=	5'guanosine monophosphate
PDE5	=	phosphodiesterase type 5
GTP	=	guanosine triphosphate
NO	=	nitrous oxide
NANC	=	non-adrenergic/non-cholinergic fibres

Figure 5.1: Intracellular process controlling erection.

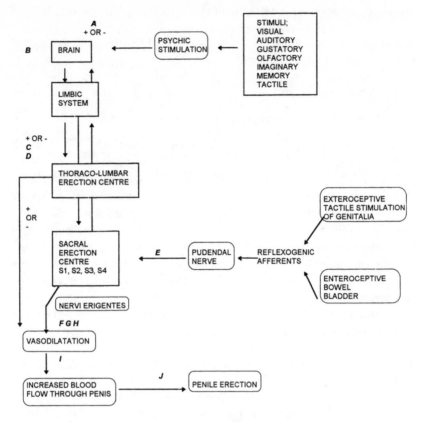

EXPLANATION OF TEXT

A   Psychological factors are among the most common factors for erectile dysfunction.

B   Lesions in the anterior temporal lobe (vascular, traumatic, etc.)

C   Complete suprasacral spinal cord lesion, which permits only reflexogenic erection.

D   Incomplete suprasacral spinal cord lesion, which allows erection of either reflexogenic or psychogenic origin.

E   Complete infrasacral spinal cord lesion, which abolishes erection.

F   Autonomic neuropathy leads to impotence (such as diabetes).

G   Radical pelvic surgery can cause damage to the local nerve plexus (such as abdominoperineal resection of the rectum.

H   Drugs that inhibit the action of acetylcholine.

I   Major vascular occlusion in the abdomen or pelvis, which impedes blood supply to penile tissue.

J   Fibrous plaque of Peyronie's disease and damage to the cavernous tissue after prolonged priapism can be a major problem.

In addition, many endocrine disorders are associated with impotency (for example hypopituitarism, Addisons disease, adrenal feminization), but the mechanism remains unclear.

Figure 5.2: Causes of erectile dysfunction (adapted from Tomlinson, 1999).

Improving Erectile Ability

The commonest method of producing erection is through the injection of drugs directly into the tissues of the penis. Until the late 1980s the three most common drugs used were papaverine hydrochloride, phenoxybenzamine and phentolamine, more recently followed by prostaglandin E-1 (PGE-1), vasoactive intestinal polypeptide (VIP) and thymoxamine.

Papaverine acts as a nonspecific antispasmodic which relaxes all smooth muscles containing structures. While papaverine may be considered the classic drug of choice, it is not without complications. Priapism (prolonged erection) may occur; if overdosed upon it may induce acute cardiovascular reactions and hypotension; and some fibrosis of the tissue area most frequently used for injection has also been reported. Due to these side effects and the evidence of the efficacy of other drugs, the use of papaverine appears to be on the decline in the able bodied population (Junemann *et al.*, 1991), but is still advocated for those with spinal cord injury (Yarkony *et al.*, 1995).

Phenoxybenzamine is a potent alpha-adrenoceptor antagonist (AAA) used as an oral agent in the treatment of arterial hypotension. Despite its potency in inducing erection it is not recommended, both because of its extremely long half life and because it binds to receptors on cell surfaces. Phentolamine is another AAA, but it also blocks serotonin receptors and has effects which are reversible. It is ineffective taken orally but in combination with papaverine, PGE-1 or VIP is highly effective. Both thymoxamine and VIP are still subject to clinical evaluation, leaving PGE-1 as the most extensively tested newer drug.

PGE-1 occurs naturally in many parts of the body including the cavernous tissue of the penis. It is synthesized under the generic name alprostadil and marketed as Prostin VR (Upjohn medical) and Prostavasin (Schwarz-Pharma, Germany). It is registered for use in congenital heart disorders in newborn children and in peripheral arterial disease. It relaxes penile smooth muscle that has been precontracted with either prostaglandin F2 alpha or norephedrine and when injected into the corpora in the penis produces erection. More recent developments allow for delivery of the drug into the external meatus of the urethra (MUSE).

Systemic side effects are rare following injection and erection duration of over 4 hours, indicative of development of priapism, are rare. However, a number of able bodied men report penile pain (of unclear aetiology) when PGE-1 is injected, which often remains for the duration of the erection. Men with complete spinal cord injury rarely experience such pain but the effects of MUSE in this population have yet to be established.

Drugs may therefore not be either appropriate or acceptable to many men, particularly where some penile sensation remains. In these cases a wide variety of vacuum assistance devices may be used each of which works on the principle of encouraging engorgement of the penis by development of a partial vacuum and then constricting the outflow of blood using a ring placed at the base of the shaft. Such devices allow for erections of up to 30 minutes and may be used by individuals more frequently than drug therapy.

A more drastic approach to impotence treatment is the surgical insertion of silicone rods into the corpora which either produce a permanent erection or which can be inflated at will. The major side effects of such an approach are the risks of rejection and the lack of clarity regarding the effects of implants of this sort on denervated tissue in the longer term.

In general, most male patients opt for the use of injection therapy; those who have some sensation and who wish to engage more frequently in sexual activity than the dosage limitations allow frequently use vacuum assistance devices at other times.

Using the drug [intracavernosal injection of papaverine] *is no big deal ... I can't feel it anyway. When I've talked to male friends about it they often say they could never do that ... but I say, you're not in my situation ... think of all the men who go to impotence clinics ... what do you think they are doing? ... then they come around. The clincher is I get erections which last around an hour, my partner's never been happier, and it doesn't cost me a thing.* (Male, 28, T7 complete paraplegia)

Viagra (Sildenafil)

This drug has become one of the most commonly discussed methods of treating impotence in the twentieth century. Research into the efficacy of Viagra among the spinal cord injury population was first undertaken in the United Kingdom (Glass *et al.*, 1997c; Derry *et al.* 1998; Maytom *et al.*, 1999).

Viagra is effective as an oral therapy for erectile dysfunction due to a wide range of causes. It acts as a selective inhibitor of phosphodiesterase type 5 (PDE-5) and therefore enhances the concentration of cGMP which in turn maximizes smooth muscle relaxation in the corpus cavernosum; where men with spinal cord injury are able to obtain some erectile response to stimulation, Viagra enhances it (see Figure 5.3).

The work undertaken in the United Kingdom has shown the drug to be effective regardless of lesion level; patients with injuries above T6 (and therefore with increased risk of dysreflexia) did not experience dysreflexic episodes during the trials. Similarly, men with

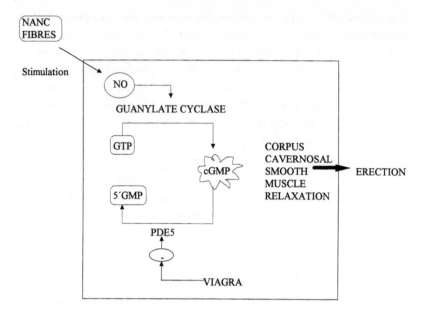

VIAGRA ACTS AS INHIBITOR OR PDE5 ACTIVITY AND ENHANCES
CONCENTRATION OF cGMP LEADING TO OPTIMALIZATION OF
SMOOTH MUSCLE RELAXATION AND ERECTION

KEY

cGMP	=	cyclic guanosine monophosphate
5'GMp	=	5'guanosine monophosphate
PDE5	=	phosphodiesterase type 5
GTP	=	guanosine triphosphate
NO	=	nitrous oxide
NANC	=	non-adrenergic/non-cholinergic fibres

Figure 5.3: Effect of Viagra on erectile dysfunction.

complete lower motor neurone damage may not benefit from using
Viagra. However, clinical experience would suggest such cases to be
rare; diagnosis of complete LMN damage requires extensive neurological examination in the context of the desire to obtain erection. Patients
with high level injuries and LMN damage should seek further opinion
from their treating clinician.

Fertility

Menstruation Following Spinal Cord Injury

Spinal cord injury for women is often associated with alteration in
menstrual patterns. Current evidence from the USA would suggest

that almost 60 per cent of women show some alteration in menstrual pattern after spinal cord injury. Over 50 per cent of this group experience secondary amenorrhea for between 3 to 6 months, and up to one year, post-injury (Yarkony, 1992). The primary cause is believed to be the impact the stresses associated with having experienced a spinal cord injury have on the pituitary–hypothalamic–ovarian axis. Once amenorrhea is stabilized, fertility for women returns to normal levels. This evidence is supported by more recent investigations of menstruation following paediatric spinal cord injury (Anderson and Mulcahey, 1997). These authors studied 37 females who were injured before their 16th birthday; 22 were injured prior to menarche, 15 post-menarche. No significant menstrual problems were noted in either group.

Semen Potency and Ejaculation

Semen potency and ejaculation are both significantly affected in men following spinal cord injury. The process of ejaculation is complex (Chapelle *et al.*, 1992) and most studies report significant reduction in both ejaculation and fertility of ejaculate following spinal cord injury. Ejaculation involves closure of the bladder neck (through sympathetic stimulation) and relaxation of the external sphincter. Patients with spinal cord injury often experience retrograde ejaculation because of sympathetic damage, and a number of processes have been attempted to induce an ejaculate.

Although erection is noted in 54–82 per cent of men, ejaculation is reported only in 3–15 per cent (more commonly in lesions that are lower motor neurone, lower in the cord, and incomplete). Similarly, fertility is reported in only 0–5 per cent of men, with lower and incomplete lesions being more fertile. However, wide individual variation prevents using lesion characteristics to predict accurately an individual person's sexual potential. Similarly, more recent research (Bennett *et al.*, 1987) would also suggest that, using appropriate electrovibratory techniques, a greater percentage of men are able to produce motile semen a number of years after their injury. At the simplest level, couples may be taught how to introduce semen, obtained with the vibrator at home, into the vagina using a standard syringe. Where semen motility is low (less than 35 per cent) in vitro fertilization (IVF) can be of benefit. More recently developed micro-assisted fertilisation techniques require only small numbers of motile sperm. Intracytoplasmic sperm injection (ICSI) is more suited for those with low sperm counts as semen is inserted directly into the egg cytoplasm. Research indicates fertilization rates as high as 70 per cent and childbirth rates as high as with IVF.

Fertility Counselling

The notion of assisted conception support following spinal cord injury therefore takes on a slightly different perspective as the induction of ejaculation is rarely a primary factor for those who are able bodied. Systems of assisted conception are not normally part of the processes of care undertaken within most spinal cord injury centres in the United Kingdom. However, in those centres where services do exist there remains the need to conform to statutory regulation. Indeed the Human Fertilization and Embryology Act (HFEA) (HFEA, 1990) places considerable emphasis on supportive counselling for those considering fertility support and there are a number of specific issues for those with spinal cord injury which must be addressed.

> *We went along to see a counsellor before Bill and I could get [fertility] treatment. This consisted of her reading from a pamphlet and us saying whether we understood or not. With hindsight there were so many issues we should have thought about but at the time all we wanted to do was have a child.*
> (Partner of male, 32, C6 complete tetraplegia)

The HFEA Code of Practice specifies three types of support which should be available to couples:

1. Implications counselling;
2. Support counselling;
3. Therapeutic counselling.

The later Kings Fund investigations (Kings Fund, 1991) recommended information counselling in addition; the comments of the above couple indicate some variability in the quality of counselling support available throughout the country.

For male patients following spinal cord injury the issue of potency is often raised soon after admission either by the person themselves or their parents. Patients often request 'a sperm test' before they leave the centre and clinicians should beware of providing this as a routine procedure for a number of reasons.

There remains the notion of 'normality' following spinal cord injury; few able bodied people know whether they are fertile or not unless they have attempted to have a child for at least 6-12 months. Indeed infertility is defined as:

The inability to conceive after 1 year engaging in sexual intercourse without conception.

Stanton and Dunkel-Schetter (1991)

and even for those who might be considered normally fertile the process of fertilization is not particularly efficient:

33% conceive within the first month of trying and between 25–35% take more than one year.

Tennen *et al.* (1991)

Individuals should be given time to re-establish their role following discharge in order that they may be given time to examine fully their motivations to assess their own fertility.

Bill: I'd asked for a sperm test after about three months [following injury] *after talking to the other men in the centre. I hadn't realized the doctor would want to talk to my girlfriend so that was a bit of a shock to her. But when he explained I realized it wasn't simply a matter of being able or not able. My girlfriend asked me after about how I'd feel if it turned out she was the one with the problems and how would that affect our relationship. Then I thought, what if I can't; will she eventually go off with someone else.* (Male, 32, C6 complete tetraplegia)

Indeed adequate preparation, comprehensive information and ongoing support to both partners is essential throughout the entire process of assisted conception.

Sally: I hadn't realized how much feelings would fluctuate. After finding out we would need to use Dave's sperm we had two cycles which failed. I'm hopeful that the present attempt will be successful but not knowing either way makes me more snappy. (Wife of male, 28, T4 complete paraplegia)

Individuals and families need time to examine how the 'new' disability affects them and their relationships, re-establish some level of intimacy and explore their capabilities to the full. Premature involvement in fertility programmes and the testing of fertility, motility and morphology should be avoided, at least until couples have had the opportunity to address issues of returning to home and work more fully.

Sexuality

Bogle *et al.* (1980) define sexuality in the following terms: 'the integration of physical, emotional, intellectual and social aspects of individual's personality expresses maleness or femaleness'. A definition of sexuality that encompasses more than genital and motor functioning is particularly important for people with disabilities, whose opportunities for purely physical interactions with the world may be limited.

> *Just because I can't move my body doesn't mean I don't get turned on or I can't turn* [him] *on. He knows from what we say, what I wear, how I smell, and how I look at him what's on my mind.* (Female, C5 sensory incomplete tetraplegia)

A person who is not able to use parts of their body or senses, or who feels or indeed does not look like other men or women, has as much right to full sexual expression as anybody else.

However, as Cole (1988) notes,

> society is still struggling with the negative concept that disabled people are asexual and could not possibly have concerns or problems regarding sexuality in the same way as able bodied people.
>
> (p. 277)

Early research looking at sexuality after spinal cord injury tended to have a physiological emphasis, concentrating for men on erectile function and fertility, and for women on reproduction and pregnancy (Higgins, 1979; Wilmuth, 1987; Baker and Cardenas, 1996), with the sexual functioning of men having been dealt with far more extensively in the literature (Zwerner, 1982; Wilmuth, 1987). This may be partly explained by the higher incidence of SCI in men than in women. However, a more significant issue is the view, essentially of male researchers, that sexual dysfunction is less traumatic for women:

> women's physical re-adjustment is less problematic because they play a passive role in sexual intercourse.
>
> (Ford and Orifier, 1967)

> *When I read that quote I thought, what the hell does he know. There is no way I'd consider my role as passive in anything, let alone sex. I don't consider myself a feminist or a politician ... just the same as everyone else ... with the same wants and skills as everyone else.* (Female, 42, C6 central cord syndrome)

106

More recently, researchers have begun to examine issues of sexual satisfaction and drive for women following spinal cord injury (Black *et al.*, 1998). When directly compared with able bodied women, SCI women showed significantly lower levels of sexual satisfaction and drive and significantly higher levels of psychological symptoms and negative affect. However, when the data were adjusted for confounding variables, married SCI women were no less sexually satisfied than able bodied women, which may reflect partner availability as the key influencing variable affecting sexual satisfaction. Given the limitations of the sample, the authors reinforce the need for further examination of both the physical and psychological factors associated with female sexual function and sexuality.

Individual variability may therefore be considered as fundamental to an expression of sexuality and sexual need as it is in all other areas of life. Within the area of spinal cord damage it is important to understand the potential differential effects of various types of disability on such expression. A congenital spinal cord disability is likely to permeate all aspects of sexual development; for example, a lack of privacy and independence in daily living may interfere with the process of acquiring sexual knowledge. Similarly, there is often considerable over-protection by families and a reluctance of clinical personnel to raise sexual issues with those below the age of consent. An acquired disability is more likely to have different implications depending on the stage of life in which it occurs. For example, acquiring a disability early in life may have diffuse effects such as the interruption of gender role and sexual development, whereas a person who acquires a disability after reaching adulthood may be more likely to recognize specific losses. There are also differences between progressive and stable conditions; for instance the uncertainty and anxiety created by a progressive disability can compromise spontaneity and forward planning.

When John was first diagnosed [progressive spinal cord tumour] *it took a while to get on with life again. It has taken a long time to take each day as it comes rather than be on the lookout every day for signs that things are getting worse.* [Questioned further regarding intimacy] *... Well that was the same ... I thought what if I get pregnant again ... would I cope as John got worse. We talked it through on lots of occasions and eventually realized we were spending so much time talking about it life was beginning to pass us by. Emma's five now, John's still with us and we have a good quality of life. If there's one thing I would say to other people it's take each day at a time. There's no point looking too far ahead and worrying yourself into an early grave.* (Wife of male, 33, spinal tumour)

More than two-thirds of relationships survive the trauma of SCI. The many changes involved in acquiring a disability can place relationships under considerable strain. Relationships for women may be particularly vulnerable when a man has to take on a caring role where the woman's role had previously been bound up with caring for a male partner (Morris, 1989). However, the number of sustained relationships goes some way in challenging the myth that people with disabilities do not have partnerships or sexual relationships.

When Rick and I said we were going to marry some people were really off. Rick told me his father had tried to talk him out of it . . . he'd said he should marry someone who could help look after him as well. We both knew what he meant and I suppose I can see it from his point of view in a way. We all get on well though . . . I think he's started to realize that we really love one another . . . I suppose men find love more difficult to cope with than women do. (Male, 24, C5 complete tetraplegia; Female, 23, T2 complete paraplegia)

In discussing the quality of their relationships, many people have stressed the need to be independent of their parents and partners, and particularly the value of open communication.

This marriage works because we have our own space. There's nothing worse than being under one another's feet all the time. It's not like we've had a row or anything . . . I just need time for me. It's like when dad retired . . . mum couldn't do what she'd done for years because he was there and it sort of threw her routine out. I promised myself even before the accident that I'd never let myself get in that situation and the accident hasn't changed my view on that. (Male, 31, L1 incomplete paraplegia)

Those with disabilities may have concerns regarding sexuality because they differ physically from those who are able bodied, or they may have been denied sex education or information; they may have questions about their role in society, about their femininity or masculinity and self-image. With increased acceptance of sexual variety and information about sexuality, an increased repertoire of sexual behaviours is indicative of a satisfying sexual relationship following injury (Bregman and Hadley, 1976; Becker, 1978; Zwerner, 1982). More attention is now paid to the psychosocial and rehabilitative aspects of sexuality, which are regarded as an essential aspect of comprehensive care, although the service remains patchy.

Recent research has indicated that although on average those with spinal cord injury report an increase in sexual dysfunction, their feelings about sex, and their consideration of which aspects of sexual activity are important, remain largely unchanged (Kreuter *et al.*, 1994a, 1994b, 1996) In particular, increases in dysfunction tend to be slight exacerbations of problems experienced prior to the injury, especially those related to arousal and climax. Aspects of love-making other than foreplay and intercourse, such as holding and touching, tend to increase in relative importance, although again there is a moderate level of variation. However, it must always be remembered that expression of generalities in such a complex field as adjustment to trauma or illness should be undertaken with caution.

When individuals are questioned about their perceptions of whether their spinal problems have affected their sex life, a number of studies show that people generally indicate their sex life has been affected for the worse, although about a quarter report no change and approximately 5 per cent of people feel that their sex life improves after injury. Although sexual relationships may well be worse, it must be remembered that there is little available evidence concerning levels of premorbid functioning.

> *Sure, on the whole things are not be the same as before the accident but I never expected them to be. We make love when we want to. It's not a competition . . . People think because they read in the* [tabloid newspaper] *that people have it fifteen times a night that that's normal . . . No way!* (Male, 59, C6 central cord syndrome)

In keeping with a broader concept of sexuality, account must also be taken of how people feel about their bodies.

> *He won't have mirrors in the house now. Occasionally he gets a sight of himself in a shop window and I can see he looks away. When I asked him why he just said he's not ready to see himself yet.* (Wife of male, 68, C4 complete tetraplegia; ventilator dependent)

In a recent study of women with spinal cord injury (Harrison *et al.*, 1995), 'overall' satisfaction was comparable to a control group of able bodied women. When measuring 'body' satisfaction, however, disabled women showed significantly greater dissatisfaction than able bodied women, although it was significantly less than that felt by those with eating disorders. Generally, dissatisfaction was found to increase with age and the level of disability, but it was not associated with sexual frequency or dysfunction. Paralysis frequently causes a loss of muscle tone in the stomach and legs; leg muscles may atrophy, and it may be difficult to avoid putting on weight around the stomach region. These effects are reported by women to account for most of their increased body dissatisfaction.

> *When I look at myself I get upset mainly with my tummy. I used to have a really flat stomach and now it just flops in front of me. I cope with it like most women do . . . I make the most of my good features . . . slap on the war paint and away I go.* (Female, 26, T7 complete paraplegia)

There remain problems in elucidating meaningful information concerning sexual practice and perceptions of sexuality with both questionnaires and interviews. Although questionnaires allow a more economical use of the researcher's time, and ensure that questions are standardized, they do not ensure that questions have been understood. There are still limits on the questions that can be asked about sex that are completely without ambiguity and the possibility of misinterpretation, especially if the wording is not to become insensitive or absurd. There is little research evidence to identify which information is best obtained by questionnaire, and which by interview; much may depend on the level of rapport or trust that can be established by an interviewer.

Feelings about sex, and the aspects of sexual activity that are considered important, essentially remain unaffected by acquired disability. There are many potential causes for the increase in reported sexual dysfunction, ranging from physical and emotional to social and financial factors. Many of the physical reasons concern impaired bowel and/or bladder function, and pain, spasms and cramp. Such issues tend not to affect desire, but rather interrupt or stop sexual activity; an increase in problems does not mean a declining interest in sex or involvement in sexual relationships. Exploration of sexuality tends to remain unmet by current clinical services; the comments of service users underlines the fact that sexuality is an important part of overall functioning. It should be remembered, however, that people with disabilities, just like able bodied people, can have sexual dysfunctions of purely psychological origin, caused by the grief response to loss, or worries about having children or financial difficulties. The effect that acquired disability can have on sexuality frequently depends on circumstances before the injury. Those with pre-injury experience of comfort and delight in sensual activity can often recover these good feelings, although the way in which loss is experienced and the kind of initial care given is very important to this process.

Earlier research (Dell Fitting *et al.*, 1978) had indicated a correlation between 'sense of attractiveness' and being in a sexual relationship. However, more recent research (Harrison *et al.*, 1995) does not show an association between body satisfaction and being in a relationship. This would suggest that body dissatisfaction/disparagement does not appear to be a key feature of 'self-image' which affects sexual adjustment. Many people have also indicated how part of dealing with their changed body shape has been to pay more attention to the head and upper body:

I was always keen on sports and getting involved with the sports club since my accident has helped me get going again. I've built up my upper body more than I ever did before and I feel good about that ... It's made me feel more confident about myself. (Female, 35, T11 complete paraplegia)

In response to a number of disabling conditions, and following surgery, changes in affect are commonly reported. In terms of anxiety, a spinal condition may represent the constant stress of coping with disability in an able bodied world. Access and transport difficulties are familiar themes raised by ex-patients

I remember being in America some years ago and found I could get on all the buses in my chair and thinking if they can do it why can't we. Have you ever tried getting into a night club or a cinema? The usual excuse is that I pose a fire risk ... maybe they think I'm going to spontaneously combust or something. I can laugh about it now but it does get me down ... What chance have I got in meeting a woman if I can't even get near them? (Male, 26, Sensory incomplete T3 paraplegia)

Similarly, depression may arise in the response to the many losses; body function, independence, choices. It is commonly reported that there is often, during rehabilitation, little acknowledgement of the emotional aspects of the person's experience. Sexuality is rarely mentioned during their care, and this is considered unhelpful. Higher levels of anxiety and depression are associated with negative feelings about sexual activity, and it may be expected that people who are depressed and anxious would also report other negative emotions. In examining association between affective state and sexual dysfunction, there remains the difficulty of establishing the causal relationship and although it is not clear which causes the other, sexual stimulation needs to be accompanied by the appropriate emotional conditions, and anxiety and fear are known to have an inhibiting effect on sexual arousal and response (Kitzinger, 1983; Katchadourian, 1990).

The insensitivity to sexual needs and lack of understanding by health professionals is also regarded by many as a hindrance to their adjustment to disability (Dell Fitting *et al.*, 1978; Zwerner, 1982). The fact that most medical professionals are able bodied and male is likely to have contributed to the particular failure to address issues of sexuality for women with disabilities, and the greater numbers of male spinal patients may also have indirectly contributed to some lack of understanding of the needs of women.

Many interviewees expressed the opinion that women patients were somehow 'left out' during hospital care, and that there was a degree of sexual stereotyping in what was expected of the male and female patients. (Research psychologist)

Principles of Psychosexual Therapy

Where systems of support exist, these should be capitalized upon. An excellent series of texts is available through the SIA which address the needs of heterosexual, homosexual and lesbian sexual relationships (Hooper, 1994a, 1994b; Hooper and Regard, 1994a, 1994b). The importance of open, honest communication is a central tenet of all self-help publications, and indeed remains so in the event of an individual's need or desire to receive psychosexual support. Society in general is becoming more enlightened to the benefits of highly trained and skilled psychological therapy, and there is an increasing acceptance of the benefits of addressing concerns and difficulties with a detached third party in a confidential setting. However, there continues to be a greater referral of those for whom difficulties had become increasingly acute rather than presentation for preventative support, as a consequence of the failure of most rehabilitation settings to subsume such discussion within their cultures. It is essentially to those who find themselves in an acute situation and wishing to seek support that this section is addressed.

The theoretical framework adopted by clinicians continues to be simply a matter of personal preference. Jehu (1979) in his book *Sexual Dysfunction* begins on a personal note by stating that he considers himself to be a behaviour therapist, not a sex therapist, as he applies essentially the same approach whether he is dealing with a sexual or any other kind of psychological difficulty.

There are numerous theoretical approaches to counselling ranging from psychotherapy, psychoanalysis, cognitive, phenomenological, and behavioural therapies. While the therapy adopted depends on the therapist's own position, what must remain central to the issue is that the applied therapy be appropriate to the *needs* of the individual. For those with physical disabilities the application of behaviourally-based therapies, within a framework based on functional analysis, has been shown to have significant benefits as it focuses on practical aspects of treatment (see Chapter 3).

When individuals first enter a clinician's door for assistance, they should be reassured that they have undertaken the most difficult step; that of accepting a difficulty exists. Whatever the cause of the problem, either through physical or psychological support, some improvement should be possible. One of the first issues which frequently needs to be addressed in therapy is the nature of the presenting difficulty. Following injury patients are more likely to attribute any change in functioning to the trauma, such that it is often difficult for patients to accept that their difficulty may not have a physical basis. In helping the patient to overcome this it is often helpful to go through each of the assessment procedures undertaken in turn, where possible showing the person the original data and explaining what each means. This may include, in the case of secondary impotence, detailed explanation of the hormone profile following blood tests, explanation of the purpose of doppler ultrasound for measuring penile pulses, or using printouts of nocturnal tumescence data to reinforce the observation of full tumescence during sleep. Patients are often concerned that referral to a clinical psychologist means they have a mental difficulty, rather than a normal reaction to an essentially rare or abnormal traumatic event.

Exploring 'physical' data and emphasis on practical solutions to difficulties during behavioural therapy serve to reinforce the 'normality' of the situation. Viewing psychological problems as learnt ways of responding in situations which are amenable to change also enables the client to begin to accept some degree of involvement or responsibility for the genesis of the condition. The inability to experience arousal, or to obtain an erection in the absence of any physical abnormality, may therefore be seen as a specific behavioural difficulty. The skill of the therapist is in enabling the client to view their sexual difficulty as a learnt behaviour and, as such, therefore amenable to change, provided the conditions which led to the difficulty are modified in some way. Related to this issue is the need to involve the partner in therapy. In sexual dysfunction it is considered that some aspect associated with the interaction while making love acts as a negative stimulus to either or both partners. It is common, for example, for women with spinal cord injury to experience severe spasms, which reduces sexual activity for fear of inducing such a difficulty. Similarly, the inability of a man with spina bifida to obtain an erection may be due in part to feelings of inadequacy, or feelings of embarrassment associated with the possibility of urine leakage.

The use of both partners in therapy is considered important, and is supported by research data from many areas of disability (Clement and Schmidt, 1983), but there are a small number of cases where the

113

sexual problem might not be seen as a relationship difficulty. The inability to function sexually due to strict moral or religious upbringing may result due to the individual never having learnt the cues or techniques involved in foreplay or love making. In one such case initial therapy was given to an individual, and was only extended to include a partner some months later, once he had become established in a stable relationship.

However, in most cases, if patients and spouses are to begin to overcome their specific psychosexual difficulty then it is important that communication is as accessible and unambiguous as possible. One of the primary aims of therapy is therefore to provide an atmosphere which is conducive to the exploration of the potential factors associated with the expressed difficulty in such a way as to provoke the least amount of anxiety for either partner.

A review of five sexual counselling programmes for people with spinal injuries (Schuler, 1982) concluded that there appeared to be a number of common factors. The initial stage of most programmes was the presentation of information regarding sexual function and the resultant changes following trauma. The examination of prejudice and the exploration of myths surrounding sexuality were approached at the same time as the information was being presented. A major goal of all programmes was for the injured person to redefine their sexuality, exploring the compensations which had to be made for the loss of function in various parts of the body, and redefinition of those areas which produced the greatest degree of arousal. As each group progressed there was an increasing emphasis placed on practical activity and an exploration of the individual's needs.

The provision of such support groups in the UK falls short of the number available in the USA. It also remains unclear whether the exploration of sexuality in a large group format is the most efficient way of disseminating information, or whether individual couple therapy enables both the therapist and those engaged in therapy to retain more control over both the pace at which issues are raised, and gives them the opportunity to refrain from discussion of personal issues related to the interaction within the couple's relationship.

Those couples who report greatest benefit from therapy are those who make a comprehensive examination of one another's behaviour in the early sessions. Similarly, those who are more receptive and committed to the assignment exercises tend to pass through therapy more quickly, though given the high degree of individual variability in both the determinants and content of the presenting difficulty, there are no set guidelines for the number of sessions required. Cooper's (1969) assertions that those cases in which the partner co-operates in therapy respond significantly better would appear to have some face validity.

Developing Psychosexual Awareness in SCI Centres

Service developments in rehabilitation continue to fall behind the needs of the service users and the best efforts of those employed within the centres (Ward and Houston, 1993), and there is a danger in overstating the medicalization of remedial sexual therapies. The experience of acceptable sexual activity and sexuality forms part of perceived quality of life (Ferrans and Powers, 1992) which involves not only an acceptable level of health and functioning, but also adjustment in psychosocial, financial and family support issues. Although there is some standardization and agreement over practice concerning treatment of secondary erectile failure, ejaculatory dysfunction and fertility, the ability and willingness of professionals to engage in exploration of sexuality, as essentially a communication exercise, remains less consistent. Close liaison must exist between a wide range of skilled therapists in order to provide comprehensive screening of physical and psychosocial correlates of every form of sexual difficulty and dysfunction. It must become the responsibility of each service discipline to establish a framework within which concepts, and indeed preconceptions and prejudices, may be explored. Training programmes provide the opportunity to explore these issues in an essentially safe and protective environment. This provides protection both to members of staff and to patients themselves.

Encouraging and enabling staff to engage in discussion of sexual topics and therapy must not be prescriptive. There is still considerable sensitivity and taboo concerning open sexual discussion. A fundamental issue which does require thought before beginning to provide psychosexual support is the therapist's own perceptions and feelings about sexual activity. Potential therapists must have a comprehensive knowledge of the literature pertaining to normal and dysfunctional activity, must examine and resolve their own prejudices, and in the field of neurological trauma and disease have a sound understanding of the physical and psychosocial implications on both the individual, the family, and their role in society. While such a statement should not need to be made, there remain numerous instances where such issues have not been resolved. Cases have often been referred to the author, after having been seen by numerous therapists where, for example, differential diagnosis (defining whether the cause is physically or psychologically based) of the presenting condition has not been attempted, or couples have been refused therapy once it became clear that they were involved in same sex relationships.

Prejudices must therefore be explored in considerable detail; those who wish to work with sexual dysfunction must be aware of their own limitations; discussing adult heterosexual activity is in itself presumptive given the increasing frequency with which same sex relationships report for psychosexual counselling; and the issues of HIV infection, preparation of both partners for fertility programmes, and dealing with negative outcomes all require considerable expertise and sensitivity.

In order that a forum may develop to expand the discussion of sexually related issues there is a need for centres to develop a philosophy of care which not only encourages open exploration, but which also ensures the provision of an adequately trained team of staff who might provide specialist support. Excluding an accepted physical basis for an expressed difficulty should not be considered as conclusive for a diagnosis of psychological aetiology; such a diagnosis must only be made on the basis of objective criteria in support of the diagnosis.

Summary

There exist a number of treatment options to enable men to obtain erection and ejaculate following spinal cord injury. Research concerning female sexual function is sparse and remains an area of essentially unmet clinical need. However, medicalization of function should be viewed with caution and must be balanced against the emotional needs of both partners and be contextually appropriate. Service developments should ensure equitability between physical and psychological support.

Whatever the therapeutic strategy adopted by investigators for the treatment of psychosexual dysfunction, what remains clear is the need for more methodologically rigorous investigation. In no field is this more true than in the assessment of those factors associated with the development and maintenance of psychosexual dysfunction in people who have congenital and acquired neurological disabilities. The use of objective assessment methods may be one way in which the efficacy of psychosexual counselling procedures may be established. There is some evidence available that day erection measurement pre- and post-treatment provides accurate measurement of improvement through biofeedback, and the design of valid and reliable questionnaires for use at similar times, and at longer term follow up, may also prove useful. Such assessment and therapeutic tools must be patient centred and there remains the need to view sexuality as part of global quality of life issues for those with neurological disability; development of wide staff awareness of need and intervention skills within physical rehabilitation settings should go some way to adequately address this problem.

Further Reading

Morris, J. (Ed.) (1989). *Able Lives: Women's Experience of Paralysis*. London: Women's Press.
Well-written and readable account of women's experiences of hospitals, community life and coping in general with spinal cord injury. Currently out of press but available through inter-library loans.

Katchadourian, H.A. (1990). *The Biological Aspects of Human Sexuality*, 4th ed. New York: Holt, Rinehart & Winston.
Excellent introduction to physiological mechanisms, effects and treatment of wide range of dysfunctions.

Sipski, M.L. and Alexander, C.J. (1997). *Sexual Function in People with Disability and Chronic Illness*. Gaithersburg, MD: Aspen Publishers.
Probably the most up-to-date reference book available on sexual function in spinal cord injury. Good review of general effects on sexual function, excellent chapter in Part II on spinal cord injury and good overviews of treatment.

6

So Is It All Worthwhile?

Permanent Ventilation and Complete Tetraplegia

Introduction

While it is recognized that there is no such thing as an 'acceptable' level of spinal cord injury, most people living with such disability accept that tetraplegia (paralysis below the neck) is probably the most devastating experience as it produces total, usually sudden, loss of control of life. Rehabilitation after such a catastrophic injury is emotionally overwhelming, financially costly, and requires a considerable length of time. Hospital treatment alone, without considering the expenses of social support, special appliances and community care, costs approximately £16,000,000 a year to the exchequer (Krishnan, 1993). Furthermore for a number of patients who experience injury above the level of C4, there is frequently the added complication of ventilator dependence, due to the neurological inability to control the diaphragm. It is these people who others would most consider to have experienced the greatest physical loss. Life expectancy has continued to improve for this group over the past 25 years, with mortality rates since 1986 reduced by over 90 per cent for those surviving over one year (DeVivo and Ivie, 1995). Recent medical advances have meant that a number of such individuals have received phrenic nerve stimulator implantation (Glen and Phelps, 1985), which has enabled them to regain some breathing control, although this is neither a universally applicable procedure nor acceptable to all people.

The Mersey Regional Spinal Injuries Centre in Southport has over the past 18 years developed an expertise in treating those with high level tetraplegia who require permanent ventilation, and in developing support services in the community. It is the purpose of this chapter to question the assumption that still prevails in the United Kingdom

118

that such severe cases require permanent institutional care and to examine the practicalities of living in the home environment with high levels of dependence. There is an increasing body of research evidence to support the cost effectiveness and impact on quality of life of returning to the home environment (Fuhrer *et al.*, 1987; Whiteneck *et al.*, 1989; Whiteneck *et al.*, 1990; Carter, 1993; Glass, 1993; Krishnan, 1993; Bach and Tilton, 1994; Glass, 1996) and this chapter explores the implications of returning home for all family members.

Home on a Ventilator

The cornerstone of this venture is the willingness of the individual and family to adapt to the alteration in circumstances. In a recent study (Gardner *et al.*, 1985) the ethics of providing ventilation for patients who experience spinal trauma resulting in tetraplegia were discussed. The views of 21 patients and families, who between 1968 and 1984 had received ventilatory support for varying periods of time, were canvassed and 18 reported that they would wish to be temporarily ventilated again in the future should the need arise, with only one patient stating a desire to be allowed to die.

Little objective evidence is currently available concerning the views of those who receive permanent ventilation and whether they or their relatives consider it would have been better to allow them to die. Similarly, the implications of spinal cord injury on family life have received little attention; Christopherson (1968) commented on the high frequency of role reversal where a male partner experiences a spinal cord injury. It had been suggested (Brag, 1977) that the families of severely disabled individuals pass through stages of adjustment which parallel those of the individuals themselves, although more recent research has argued that such stage theory concepts of adjustment are not supported by empirical evidence (Buckelew *et al.*, 1991). Hoad *et al.* (1990) have produced a retrospective examination of the views of SCI relatives who had passed through the Stoke Mandeville Spinal Injuries Centre and concluded that they have traditionally been expected to cope with little comprehensive support. Current research undertaken by the present author (Glass, 1993) has shown that provision of comprehensive information and support to individuals and families results in a significant improvement in their understanding of the goals of the rehabilitation programme.

Since 1980, over 50 high traumatic tetraplegic patients who have been discharged home from the Mersey Regional Spinal Injuries Centre have required continued ventilation. In each case, prior to discharge, the implications for the individual and on family life were discussed, and the decision to return home arrived at following comprehensive liaison with all concerned, including the patient, family, spinal unit and community/local hospital support services. The economics and practical aspects of returning a patient requiring continued ventilation to their home were the subject of a further investigation by the staff at the spinal unit and, at a financial level alone, the saving to the exchequer is almost half the cost of keeping a patient in a hospital bed, despite the high levels of care, equipment and adaptation.

In a recent investigation, the perceived value of returning home while still requiring continual ventilation, from the point of view of both the injured person and their immediate relatives, was assessed (Glass, 1992a). Further discussions with other families in similar circumstances have expanded this data set to 25 cases.

It is a measure of the dedication of the individuals and families concerned, and their desire to help others in similar situations, that they were prepared to answer a series of very personal and searching questions. In order that the confidentiality of individual views may be maintained, the responses to each of the questions (outlined in abbreviated form below) contain interpretations of the patients' and relatives' responses as general themes.

Are you glad you are still alive?
All patients and relatives reported positively to this question.

If needed ventilator again in the future, would you prefer to die?
Two of the patients commented that if the future ventilation were permanent, or was related to severe loss of cognitive functioning, then they would rather die, while all relatives would rather the person should continue to live.

Would it have been better for the family if you had died?
The general view of patients was that if they had died at the time of their accident their families would have grieved but gradually adapted. The majority also considered that their families would have had a better quality of life if they had died, but when questioned further found it difficult to give examples. Relatives were somewhat pragmatic, stating that they would have been better off in terms of freedom to engage in other activities. There was some difficulty resolving the issue of allowing others to care for the patient against their own needs to take some respite. They often reported feeling guilty that they could not cope without assistance, although when assistance was offered within the home they became anxious that the person would not be properly cared for. Respite within the hospital was viewed favourably as it overcame these worries.

Are there any circumstances where a patient should be allowed to die?
Most respondents felt that at the time of the injury, the patient and relatives have no option but to allow life to continue as it is taken out of their hands by the hospital services. They felt that the patient should at least have the opportunity to discuss the issue while in hospital. All felt that it must always be an individual decision and therefore legislation would be difficult to impose, although in cases where there was no family support, or if there was severe associated brain trauma, that there should be an option for the person to be allowed to die.

Should just the doctor decide to ventilate?
All patient and relatives felt that the relatives should be involved to some degree in making the original decision to ventilate wherever possible, although accepted that in emergency procedures this was often not feasible. However, if the doctor had all the available information concerning the likely future for the individual then most patients would be happy for them to make the decision without family consultation.

Is there an appropriate time for the patient to decide on continuation of ventilation?
All patients felt that there were times when they wanted their ventilators switched off. These times tended to coincide with periods of physical complications, when they felt emotionally low, and when they had reached a particular plateau in their therapy. When questioned further it became clear that patients and relatives were more concerned about there being a forum within which to raise these essentially negative feelings; all commented that once they had talked the issue through they felt more agreeable to continuing ventilation.

If you experienced future complications leading to brain injury: continue ventilation?
All patients and relatives stated that if the brain injury was severe they would wish to have the ventilator turned off. The severity of the brain injury was the important factor, with patients tending more than relatives to qualify their answers by saying that if they could not communicate or enjoy activities such as reading and watching things around them, then they would rather die. Only one patient felt a desire to continue regardless of their neurological state.

If such complications occurred at the time of injury would you rather have been allowed to die?
As above, all patient and relatives felt it would be dependent upon the severity of the brain injury.

What makes life worth living for you?
Patients and relatives stated unanimously that the major factor which kept each of them going was the quality of the relationship with their family and friends. Without this degree of communication and contact most felt there would be little reason to carry on. All respondents similarly raised the issue of activity levels continuing essentially as before their accident though with a degree of compromise in some of the activities they were involved in (most notably sporting activities).

What about when your family are no longer able to look after you?
There appears to be a tacit understanding within families that should the primary care providers become unable to continue providing care, then the younger generations of family members will take over. This is true both for those who are in older age groups where the partner provides care, and for the younger patients where the siblings will provide care in the event of parental incapacity. When questioned further, most patients stated that institutional care would be tolerated but that this would not be undertaken out of choice. All patients commented that they felt fortunate to have at least spent some of their post-injury lives with their families.

How would you describe your feelings about continued ventilation?
Approximately half the patients felt that they had not really noticed the ventilator during the early stages of rehabilitation, while the other half felt some relief that it allowed them to continue to breathe. As time continued a number developed some hostility to their continued need but then settled into a routine, and no longer worried about it.

The limitations of interview procedures, and the bias attributable to 'known' investigator involvement are accepted in extending the above comments to the wider spinally injured population. However, the responses of this group as a whole tend to reflect earlier findings in the USA (Whiteneck *et al.*, 1985) that the majority of individuals report that they are 'glad to be alive since injury' and rate their quality of life as average or above. Such individuals intermittently express a wish to die, and in the present study it is notable that this group would only wish to consider death if their cognitive abilities deteriorated considerably. It is a tribute to the fortitude of the individuals concerned and the dedication of close family members that the wish to die does not occur with greater frequency. It is interesting to note the comments of one patient, who felt that at the point at which the decision to ventilate is taken, the absence of close family should be a considered factor.

The Choice to Live or Die

The ethical decisions concerning continuation of ventilation are difficult to resolve (Purtillo, 1986), though must take into account the individual's competency and informed decision to decline medical involvement. In accepting any individual for rehabilitation the primary goal must be achieving the highest level of quality of life. Implicit in such a statement is the involvement of the individual in deciding the parameters of quality, which may alter as the implications of the disability alter. As Maynard and Muth (1987) conclude:

> The ability to support a responsible choice to end life is thus consistent with, if not central to, humanistic rehabilitation.
> (Maynard and Muth, 1987: 864)

The individual's relationship with the ventilator tends to reflect the views of other trauma groups who require attachment to machinery for continued existence; haemodialysis patients often report a 'honeymoon period' when the machine is seen in an extremely positive light, followed by some swing towards rejection and then gradual acceptance (Glass *et al.*, 1987). The current trauma group, however, tended not to remember or experience the early acceptance of the ventilator due to the severity of their medical condition at this time. The anxieties experienced by relatives concerning the role of others in care reflects the need for centres who offer ventilator programmes to ensure the availability of 24-hour support and regular respite. The involvement of the family at all stages of rehabilitation, and individually tailored training programmes go some way to alleviate such anxieties, although the need for ongoing dialogue cannot be stressed too highly.

It would be wrong to attempt to extrapolate the views and experiences of this group to others requiring ventilation as they are undoubtedly a highly select population, with clear lines of communication and stable family interaction patterns. The decision to return an individual to the community must take place following comprehensive assessment of all the relevant individual medical and psychosocial factors.

In examining affective state it might be expected that the pressures of coping, on both patients and relatives, would lead to severe difficulties. This was not shown to be the case with this group of patients. In only a small number of cases were patients' depression scores above those of the normal population; similar elevated anxiety scores were only shown in three cases. There is some evidence to indicate that those who had been at home the shortest period of time experienced elevated anxiety scores, while those who had been at home longer produced higher depression scores. It is possible that patients who have been at home for short periods of time remain anxious because they are still unsure about their daily protocol and have concerns about the long-term feasibility of the arrangements, while patients who have been at home longer develop higher levels of depression because of some worries over the repetitive nature of their existence. There is certainly evidence of similar trends in other areas of loss (Glass *et al.*, 1987) for such responses to long-term illness, though the numbers involved in this study do not allow firm conclusions to be drawn. A more recent comparison of ventilator dependent patients in the UK and USA with those who had received phrenic pacers indicated higher levels of depression in the former group and higher anxiety in the latter group (Glass *et al.*, 1996). Such responses are compatible with behavioural correlates of anxiety as a form of conditioned suppression being incompatible with depression as a sudden loss of a major source of reinforcement. That patients with phrenic pacers experience higher levels of anxiety may relate either to the fact that they tend to have been injured longer (and been ventilated prior to phrenic implantation) or that there are some as yet undefined concerns regarding the long-term viability of the implants. In the related field of renal transplantation, dialysis and transplant patients have been shown to exhibit comparable affective reactions (Glass *et al.* 1996) to the latter group in response to their concerns over failure of the donor kidney after having been in place for a number of years.

Effects on the Family

Patients' perceptions of the qualities within their families indicate a high level of interaction, clarity of communication, expressiveness, high levels of organization and significantly lower levels of conflict. These perceptions correlate highly with the importance their other family members attach to good internal relationships and well-organized systems within the home. Such views also support the view of staff members that high quality of family interaction is imperative for successful community management. Similarly, the importance attached to a high level of organization within the household is understandable given the need for family members' involvement in a number of medical and caring procedures, such as maintaining the ventilator and managing the physical conditions associated with the spinal trauma.

Each family's views of the patient similarly reflect their high level of cohesion as an important factor in maintaining the family structure.

The expressed importance of the need for independence, and the need to achieve, emphasizes each family's acceptance of the injured person's need to maintain a high level of personal growth, which in itself reflects positively on all family members' desires to maintain as normal a family life as possible. As with the patients' responses, the families reflected the need for clarity and organization in maintaining the ventilator dependent person at home.

Given the essential interdependence and intensity of the relationship between the patient and family it is reassuring to see that the fundamental factor which underlines all the responses noted above is the perceived importance of a high quality of communication; the availability of good lines of communication increases the possibility for resolution of internalized concerns or distress. The availability of such open lines of communication helps militate against some of the commonly held misconceptions concerning the effects of spinal injury. It had been hypothesized that the higher the level of spinal injury, the lower the degree of emotional expression (Hohman, 1966). The comments expressed above do not support this view. Similarly, levels of motivation and achievement orientation may be expected to decline in those with severely disabling conditions, as the physical constraints reduce the range of available activities and interests. This is definitely not the case with the present group of patients and families, and has implications for ensuring access to comprehensive vocational retraining support, similar to a scheme organized in conjunction with the technical college in Southport (Fraser and Holmes, 1990).

Patients and relatives who elect to return home with ventilation are a highly selective group. There will always be the fear of complications and concerns over each individual's ability to cope. However, it is the experience in Southport that with comprehensive family, hospital and community based support, the quality of life for those requiring continued ventilation can be optimized and community reintegration should be the norm rather than the exception.

Managing Return to the Community: Case Management

In order that community reintegration may be effected, central co-ordination of the entire process is essential. There is the need to fully understand the individual circumstances of each patient and to liaise with community social services and health care purchasers and providers to ensure needs and service provision are matched. As shown in Chapter 1, the level of specialization of care which spinal injuries centres provide has arisen out of clinical need, and levels of expertise and support provided within such centres, and it remains questionable whether generic rehabilitation centres would possess either the expertise or experience to avoid the range of complications which inadequate management of such cases is likely to present. From the perspective of patients at least, the problems of longer journey times and some hardship, posed by travel to regional centres, was reported as a price worth bearing. There remain justifiable pressures on specialist centres to provide evidence of value and efficacy, and if such facilities are to continue to develop they must take radical steps to promote quality care which enables patients to maximize their rehabilitation potential. Two such developments have been fundamental to the establishment of this proposal.

Care and support systems need to be flexible to the changing needs and demands of those whom they aim to support, irrespective of age. It is with degenerative trauma that the appointment of an individual responsible for co-ordinating care may be viewed as particularly relevant and this has often been seen as the role of the family practitioner. In all rehabilitative settings, the appointment of a care co-ordinator or case manager is paramount in order to provide continuity of care, but the appointment of a case manager alone is of little relevance unless accompanied by a change in organizational philosophy and practices of care. Case management initiatives need to be applied in rehabilitation centres together with a revolving door care philosophy; patients are more likely to take on the daunting prospect of coping with life alone and, indeed, so are relatives (in the case of severely disabled patients) if they have the knowledge that immediate support is available at all times of need. The case manager should therefore maintain overall executive responsibility for rehabilitative care and admission planning, and act as the liaison point with all community services. This devolves responsibility for admission and discharge away from medical officers, who themselves must feel comfortable with the integrity and quality of the case manager. Those registered should be able to contact their centre 24 hours a day and receive advice, assistance in obtaining local services, or an appointment to see any member of the rehabilitation team (or indeed be admitted) within a time scale decided by the seriousness of the enquiry. Earlier work in Southport (Krishnan *et al.*, 1991) established functional improvement goals by which expected rehabilitation paths for specific lesion levels were established and compared on a regular basis with attainment. Regular clinical auditing, as part of the case management initiatives, has enabled the rehabilitation team to reduce inpatient rehabilitation time by, on average, 10 days, and to modify treatment schedules to reduce inpatient stay in specific conditions. For example, use of greater community surveillance and conservative management at home enabled the centre to reduce, over a five year period, both the frequency and duration of admissions for those who had developed pressure sores.

A number of initiatives to improve communication have been established in the National Health Service to encourage such developments, including the system of key workers and named nurses for individual admissions and case management initiatives. While the former have so far met with limited success, Hunter (1988) highlighted the development of case management initiatives for three client groups: an elderly population, a head injury service and a spinal injuries unit. Each was funded by the King Edward's Hospital Fund for London (The Kings Fund). The main conclusions drawn from the three sites were the importance of defining the role expectations of the case manager from the outset and a clear definition of their role in the organizational structure. Furthermore the service should provide a forum for client advocacy and ensure independence in the post; being aligned to one professional group was not seen as beneficial. Although such schemes are still in the early stages of development in the UK, the principles underlying such a service met with universal approval in the three pilot sites reported by Hunter.

Planning for discharge and the likely needs of each individual is a complex process and one which needs to take into account their particular physical, psychosocial and financial situation. A number of frameworks have been developed to assess progress through rehabilitation (see Chapter 3), and recent attempts have been made to use vocational assessment for those with spinal cord injuries. Life care planning (LCP) involves production of a comprehensive document which defines post-discharge needs as an extension of care management initiatives. This provides a costing of all physical, social and personal care support requirements and is of particular benefit in litigation cases where settlements must take account of the individual's needs throughout life.

So Has It All Been Worthwhile? A Consumer's View

It would be disingenuous for a clinician, who has a vested interest in arguing that the services he provides are indeed of value to the service user, to answer such a question. Instead, the final words must go to a man and his wife, after his recent return home on a ventilator.

Mr A: At first sight 'what is it like to be on domiciliary ventilation?' would seem to be a very simple question to answer. In doing so one has to weigh up the balance of the advantages and

127

disadvantages in relation to hospital and home. I suppose it might be possible to make out a case for spending the rest of one's life in a hospital bed, visited occasionally by friends and relatives and to be attended to by an ever changing nursing staff who are trained never to become sympathetically or emotionally involved with their patient. This prospect to me, and I suspect others, is frightening. The idea of ever-creeping institutionalism, of having very few people to talk to and the high point of every day to watch Neighbours *on television, is chilling. I became aware of the losses I was suffering at a very early stage: lack of individuality, lack of self-respect, loss of personal identity and loss of any form of intellectual stimulation.*

For me, never having been a creature of habit or routine, hospital life was a virtual nightmare with its structures, systems and regulations, all of which I readily understand, but which made life debilitating and for the most part distressing.

Perhaps I was fortunate that prior to transfer to Southport I was mostly in a coma which while in itself is not a pleasant prospect, at least relieved me of all the pain and tedium which my condition had inflicted upon me. I remember two episodes of consciousness; the first when I was told the tracheostomy had been inserted; the second, more startling, when I recalled in a hazy way that my parish priest was giving me the Last Rites. I was more than a little concerned, although not frightened, but as a Yorkshireman I remember saying to myself, 'I'm damned if I'm going to die in Lancashire.'

I have pondered long and hard as to why the Lord gave me this second chance. Certainly it has been slow, it has been very painful, but there must have been a reason, a reason which I still search for. I was lucky to be one of the few who were selected to spend time in rehabilitation in Southport. I remember, when I first arrived, all the things I could not do. I could not eat and was therefore fed through a tube; I had no sensation of taste; I could not get out of bed; I could not speak; I was totally incontinent and suffered acute spasticity. Within a week of admission to Southport I was speaking and within two had begun to eat. Being lifted daily into a wheelchair and other changes in care gradually made my life more tolerable and manageable. The greatest of these was the installation of a Baclofen pump which virtually cured my spasticity within 24 hours.

The long haul then began to enable me to return home. I am aware that purchasing authorities are often shocked that a client, as we

128

are now called, could be cared for in their own home. I was one of the lucky ones in that my Health Authority, once the financial and practical sense of the approach had been explained, supported the assembly of a care team who would look after me 24 hours a day. I remember being amused, and yet accepting the seriousness of the situation, to find that a ward of six patients would have two nurses but that I, as an individual, would have a veritable chorus-line of seven remarkably attractive young women, all at about half the cost of maintaining me in hospital. There never was a programme devised in the NHS which made more sense than this. Everyone benefits: bed space is made available, the client is at home with family, cared for to the highest possible standard, and with an umbilical cord link to the spinal unit who are able to provide instantaneous help and advice at any time of the day or night.

When the day of returning home arrives, I should imagine most people are as euphoric as I was. It is assumed that everything is suddenly going to become easier; but of course this is not the case and I had to come to terms with the fact that, apart from the location, very little had changed. I had never before experienced the kind of emotional upset which followed within a few days of my returning home. The past, at this point gave me no concern, but I found the future a most terrifying prospect, which had nothing to do with being ventilated. The hospital established milestones for progress which, upon return home, became blurred and more a personal responsibility to establish. Not knowing what the future held meant my ability to establish such goals was limited. Personally, I count myself fortunate that I have never been particularly sporting. Therefore these things I do not miss. Most of my professional life was concerned with creative and intellectual activity and this will continue.

One of the things which was not immediately apparent upon returning home is the fact that, if the mind can be so tuned, there are untold opportunities which could not have been realized in the hospital. It is sooner or later necessary to become aware of these possibilities and challenges and to try to formulate plans and methods by which they may be achieved. In other words to try to recapture ambition and drive. No easy matter, but given the support of carers family and friends, given love and encouragement, the feelings of hopelessness have a good chance of being overcome. If I answer the original question, 'what's it like to be a domiciliary ventilated person?' – well, it's not as good as being in *perfect health, but it's not so bad and a lot better than the alternative.*

Mrs A: *My husband is ventilated yet I really cannot imagine what it is like. I have thought about it endlessly, tried to imagine it in the middle of the night, learnt all about it, and yet the more I know the less I understand. It is impossible to know or comprehend the reality of paralysis and ventilation. The one thing I do know is that it is infinitely better to be ventilated at home than ventilated and living in hospital.*

Human nature being what it is, we have mercifully short memories. And now, a mere two and a half years after my husband's initial struggle to stay alive, I deal with the everyday necessities of ventilation. I even have the jargon off pat – the vent, the bag, negative pressure, etc., etc. But it is good to look back and remember for two reasons: first, it does help to put day-to-day hiccups into perspective, and second, perhaps it can give the rest of us an insight into the way people perceive someone who is ventilator dependent.

It is obvious to those families involved that someone who is ventilated is able to live at home with family and friends. Such benefits are not restricted to the patient and family, but extend to carers and the wider community.

It was only at the time of my husband's transfer that for the first time I was treated like a real person. My hopes and fears were discussed, I learnt about my attitudes to my husband's problems and how to come to terms with many of my fears. I started to see the possibility of a reasonable lifestyle emerging and as my husband became stronger his personality gradually reformed and re-emerged.

As the time approached to go home it became apparent that this was not the end in itself which it had seemed but a new and difficult beginning. What's it like to live with someone on domiciliary ventilation? It changes all the time and I am still unsure whether the changing is part of a settling in process [the person has now been at home almost two years] *or whether it will always change. The return from hospital to home is a shock to the system which one is not prepared for. The initial emotional stress and frustrations are enormous. Everywhere you go that you used to go with your partner is an upset for you. Everything he sees that he could do before and cannot do now is a slap in the face.*

Life has changed totally. We have both been changed by our suffering and our experiences and yet we want to recapture our previous relationship and our previous enjoyment of each other and our life together. The whole process of evolving an attitude to a new lifestyle is long and complicated, and probably never ends. Adjustment moves in waves, with setbacks in between. There is a whole new area of discovery while there are major practical restrictions to activity. Ventilation is exhausting in itself so additional energy has to be conserved and used wisely; making the most of opportunity is so important.

I feel life would be impossible without the care package, though I understand that some people may view the situation of people in their own home differently. Life can only be enjoyed if the ventilated person is fit and healthy within the limitations of their disability, and maximizing potential and achieving and controlling as much as possible for themselves. It is easy for the day to day necessities of healthy living to expand to fill the whole day. This is a danger and can lead to lack of confidence or stimulation and depression. Routine can be a major drag if it was not something that was previously enjoyed and lack of spontaneity can be a frustration. However, within this framework an enormous amount is achievable. Computer technology ever increases opportunities for work, entertainment and communication, and friends are an invaluable stimulation. The house allows a satisfactory and individual lifestyle to emerge in a way which it never could even in the best run hospitals.

When establishment at home with a care package is first mooted, you may be so delighted with the prospect of returning home that you will accept anything and anyone to get there as quickly as possible. In my opinion this is wrong. You can put up with most things for a few weeks but this will be for life. The close involvement, therefore, of the patient and relatives in the selection of carers and the organizational details is essential. It is worthwhile considering what you expect from them and what they expect from you. In our case we expect kindness, consideration, efficiency and enthusiasm. We receive so much more; commitment, ingenuity, support and friendship. We are very fortunate indeed, but I suspect part of the reason for this is that we all chose each other carefully in the first place.

I think the carers also expect, and hope for, certain things from us. Respect and consideration as individuals and a comfortable working environment. I recognize that I have a responsibility to try to create a positive atmosphere in the home and set an example in terms of attitude and direction. This is sometimes a tall order when I feel tired, fraught or generally off-colour, but on those occasions they make allowances for me. We all recognize that working in a sometimes highly charged home environment is not always easy, but it beneficial to consider how dreadful the alternatives are.

I said in the beginning that domiciliary ventilation was good for the patient, the relatives, carers and the community. The carers come from many different backgrounds. They have pursued their interests and beliefs by taking courses in massage, introducing us to reflexology, relaxation therapy for pain management, and many other exploits. They enjoy visiting our friends at home and in restaurants, and helping my husband with his work.

In our local community we are something of a talking point. All the carers are asked about what the job and situation is like; surely this is good – people often find it difficult asking my husband and I to our faces, and the process in some way improves their understanding of the problems faced by those with disabilities. Perhaps the next time they walk up to the top of the local hill and take a deep breath, they appreciate just how fortunate they are.

I sometimes forget the effect we have on other people. We are essentially a small band with a shared responsibility. When in Southport, our presence is the norm; out there in the real world we are perhaps quite shocking. We have a friend who tells us her relative keeps asking after my husband. When I invited her to ask this relative to visit, while she raised one concern about whether he would be in bed, the real concern which came out was whether my husband would experience a fit in her presence. A valid question. We know what we are like but we are unusual. Many people associate disability with brain damage, stroke and degenerative diseases, not with someone healthy in body and mind except for an inability to move or breathe.

It has been estimated that at the present time some 30,000 people in hospital with various disorders could be treated and living at home and that by the year 2000 this number will have increased to 100,000. The consequences for hospital and conventional nursing home accommodation and community care are significant. The use of trained lay carers in the community will surely become even more important.

Living with a ventilated person is a way of life. It requires all the skills available to you in a previous way of life. It is maddening, frustrating, frightening, exhilarating, stimulating and enriching. It is marvellous to be able to live in your own home with the person you love surrounded by the help of a good caring team.

Summary

Those who experience spinal trauma at and above the level of C4 often require continued ventilation to keep them alive. The Mersey Regional Spinal Injuries Centre in Southport has the greatest level of expertise in Europe and regularly accepts such individuals. Over the past 15 years considerable expertise has been developed in not only successfully treating almost 50 such cases, but also returning them to their home environment with full ventilator support.

Little objective evidence had been available concerning the views of those who receive permanent ventilation and whether they or their relatives consider it would have been better to allow them to die. This chapter has examined the perceived value of returning home while still requiring ventilation, from the point of view of both the injured person themselves and their nearest relatives. Although there is some alteration in affective state experienced in the majority of families, the most important factors associated with adaptation appear to be the level of communication within the family and the degree of commitment to the process shown by all family members.

Their experiences reflect the wider implications of living with disability for all those with spinal cord injuries. It would be unrealistic to suggest every injured person copes ideally; coping, by definition, is a process of getting on with life despite the desperate situations life presents. Each person, at the point of trauma, presents a unique set of personal, functional, and social circumstances to the clinical team. Providing the appropriate and timely input to a multidimensional framework, within which an individual's needs may be met throughout their life following their disability, represents the ultimate clinical challenge.

Further Reading

DeVivo, M.J. and Ivie, C.S. (1995). Life expectancy of ventilator-dependent persons with spinal cord injuries. *Chest, 108,* 1, 226–232.
Good review of available literature and authors' own research concerning the increasing life expectancy of ventilator dependent patients in the community.

Maynard, F.M. and Muth, A.S. (1987). The choice to end life as a ventilator dependent quadriplegic. *Archives of Physical Medicine and Rehabilitation*, 68, 682–684.
Thought provoking and well-written article outlining a specific case where desire to end life was addressed by the American courts.

Whiteneck, G.G. (1989). Long term outlook for persons with high quadriplegia. In G.C.Whiteneck, C. Adler, and R.E. Carter (Eds) *The Management of High Quadriplegia*. New York: Demos.
This whole book, and Whiteneck's article in particular, summarizes the available research literature and prevailing level of understanding concerning management of high level spinal cord injuries.

7

Looking Forward

Introduction

Throughout the past 50 years there has been considerable growth in understanding, treatment and support of the effects of spinal cord injury. Life expectancy, for even the most severely injured, has been extended considerably and is now almost comparable to that which might be expected by the able bodied population. At the time of the approaching new millennium, it is appropriate to assess what recent developments are likely to impact upon routine clinical practice in the near and not so distant future. This chapter summarizes the current and potential developments in care and quality of life improvement for those with SCI, and which may influence their lives in the 21st century.

Physical Science

With the advent of more comprehensive *neuroimaging techniques* it is rapidly becoming the norm for centres in the UK to have routine access to computerized tomography (CT) and magnetic resonance imaging (MRI). The improvements in technology alone are likely to make availability easier and costs lower; the associated research advances in interpretation and examination of spinal cord injury are likely to lead to further advances in knowledge of the pathologies of the cord and some application to improving diagnosis and prognosis (Boudurant, 1990). Positron emission tomography (PET) and single proton emission computed tomography (SPECT) are rapidly advancing from a research focus and are soon likely to begin to have direct bearing on routine examination of blood flow and metabolic changes in the spinal cord. The high cost and the scarceness of the equipment necessary to conduct the assessment are additional restrictive factors (Marrett *et al.*, 1988).

Functional neuromuscular stimulation (FNS), particularly important in establishing arm function for those with injuries C5 and above, is likely to develop further over the next 10 years. High tetraplegia results in significant loss to the person concerned. The principal loss of upper arm and hand function significantly reduces the independence of the individual. At the present time, surgical intervention is possible in those where lesion level is below C6. In such patients muscles innervated by the C6 segment are available for transfer to improve function. However, for those with lesions above C6, there is no scope for conducting reconstructive surgery to improve hand function, as appropriate muscles are not available for transfer. In this group of patients the only option is to implant a neuromuscular system to improve hand function.

Modern technological advances and decades of research into neuro-muscular function electrical stimulation systems have now made it possible for such a multichannel receiver/stimulator to be developed. Presently, the only system agreed by the Federal Drug Administration as suitable for such innovative work is the Neurocontrol Free Hand System (Keith *et al.*, 1989; Smith *et al.*, 1987). The implantation technique has been developed in the USA (Kilgore *et al.*, 1995a) and the surgical expertise necessary for this procedure is now available within the UK. At the time of writing, only one case has been undertaken in the UK, and further work is required on the long-term viability and efficacy of the process. The pioneering work in this area has been undertaken within Case Western University under the direction of Professor Hunter-Peckham. The unit has now assessed the results of implanting this system in five patients and the results are globally encouraging (Kilgore *et al.*, 1995b).

Orthosis

Considerable research knowledge similarly exists concerning the use of functional electric stimulation (FES) in facilitating limb function (Barbenel, 1992). The major complications at present include the inability to apply a graded stimulation (in order to replicate normal movement), and fatigue. Studies continue to develop more sophisti-cated control systems and recent research grants have been awarded to examine the possibility of multiple muscle implanted stimulation units.

However, it may be considered that the multifaceted nature of acceptance of disability is also reflected in the area of acceptance and compliance with clinical advice for the use of orthotic devices (Frederico and Renshaw, 1990; Quellete, 1991; Naylor and Mullay, 1991; Lyles and Munday, 1992; Cheng *et al.*, 1993; Doll and Michael, 1994). Patients' adherence to advice and treatment is often affected by cognitive and emotional factors operating at the point at which recommendations are received:

(a) Patients forget much of what they are told, instruction and advice are more likely to be forgotten than other information, and the more the patient is told the more they are likely to forget.
(b) Patients remember (i) what they are first told and (ii) what they consider most important.
(c) Intelligent patients do not remember more than those who are less intelligent, nor are there differences between the amount of information remembered by elderly and younger patients.
(d) Moderately anxious patients remember more than those who are highly anxious or report no anxiety.
(e) The more clinical knowledge the patient has the more they will recall. (See Cassata *et al.*, 1982.)

A number of presentational factors (Ley, 1982; Parrish, 1986) and behavioural methods (Epstein and Cuss, 1982; Haynes, 1982) have been shown to successfully enhance compliance, but the social and emotional support in the patient's environment have been shown to exert a major influence on adherence (Peck and King, 1985). Family and friends who are committed to the regime have considerable influence over promoting compliance (Rosenstock, 1985).

Providing goals and expectations for progress is an essential part of any orthotic programme but, as the information above highlights, they must take into account the specific circumstances of the individual. There are a number of models of compliance which may be applied. In practice those which have most effect are all based on a synthesis of the following:

1. Those physical, personal and situational variables which the individual brings to the rehabilitation process;
2. The processes themselves which the individual might reasonably be expected to achieve; and
3. The net beneficial effect of engaging in such processes on the individual.

The decisions, of providers and recipients, of who receives complex orthotic or implantable systems often remains a self-selecting process; on the basis of clinical knowledge of a likely candidate, the individual is approached and negotiation undertaken. While this may indeed be an appropriate process, greater knowledge and understanding of the factors to which successful, and indeed unsuccessful, acceptance and adherence may be attributed is long overdue.

Spinal regeneration

A number of models to explore the potential use of neural transplants to overcome the loss of intrinsic and extrinsic spinal neurones have been developed (Horvat, 1992) and animal experiments using embryonic neurones (as substitutes for lost or deficient host neurones) and autologous peripheral nerve segments (useful in encouraging axonal regrowth) for studying central nervous system plasticity and repair are progressing. At the present time developing the key for neural regeneration remains the 'Holy Grail' for many researchers in this area. Work is being undertaken to establish the genes which control growth and cell differentiation (Raisman, 1987). It is postulated (Kakulas, 1999) that the cure for spinal cord injury would involve enabling post-trauma expression of the genes responsible for the

> multiplication of neuroblasts, sprouting of neurites and regrowth of axons and collaterals with the restoration of physiological connections and functionally useful reflexes by means of guided plasticity and synaptogenesis.
> (Kakulas, 1999), cited in Harris (1999) p. 33.

Axon regeneration fails in the central nervous system because the glial environment is inhibitory (David and Aguayo, 1981) and it is the removal of this effect which is essential to regeneration. Fawcett (1998) and Kakulas (1999) have both reviewed a number of successful strategies which have so far been successful in animal models at lowering the functional level of loss at time of induced injury. While the benefits to those newly injured in the future may be great, there is limited understanding of the eventual possibility of such regeneration in those with long-standing spinal cord injury. While science may hold out the possibility of future regeneration, care must be given in raising too high the hopes of those presently so injured.

Prevention

Although acute care and rehabilitation remain the primary activities of spinal cord injury centres, there is a fundamental need to reduce incidence. In all areas of health care and disease there is a need to understand the process of development through which avoidance strategies may be developed. The process of health care delivery tends to be through three progressive areas of control. Primary control over health addresses issues of health promotion and specific health protection as ways in which disease and trauma may be prevented. The onset of disease or disability moves the person on to secondary control where early detection and effective treatment constitute a cure of the presenting problem. It is then only through the development of further complications or implications of the condition that people move through into tertiary control such as rehabilitation or continued and terminal care. Such a progression is dependent on a number of predisposing factors related to biology/genetics, lifestyle, environmental and health service issues, the interaction of which may be additive or multiplicative.

In combining these methods of service delivery, the importance of preventative measures for reducing personal and financial cost to both the individual and health care funding agencies becomes increasingly clear. Health care providers on both sides of the Atlantic spend increasingly larger proportions of budget allocation on secondary and tertiary support, at the expense of developing effective primary controls.

Where primary controls are developed, significant benefits may be demonstrated. Since 1983 an awareness and accident prevention programme has been promoted from the spinal injuries units of Royal North Shore Hospital, Sydney, and the Royal Rehabilitation Centre, Ryde (New South Wales) in Australia (Yeo, 1993). The programme began with limited personnel but expanded to include a co-ordinator and five lecturers who were themselves wheelchair dependent. Through a comprehensive fund raising programme it was possible to expand the service to a budget approaching A$430,000 per annum. Following widespread lobbying and education and the production of interim findings from the study, there was a reduction of 20 per cent in incidence of injuries. This reduction was identified with the introduction of compulsory seat belt legislation, random breath testing, compulsory use of helmets by motorcyclists, and education programmes as highlighted above. The cost to the community of 100 spinal cord injuries in the target area was estimated by the author at A$150,000,000 per annum. The prevention programme costs less than $500,000, or the equivalent of 10 cents for each person in the study area. The true value and contribution of the programme, which in part meant that approximately 20 families were spared the tragedy and permanent challenge presented by paralysis, is incalculable.

Psychosocial Science

The primary aim of initial post-trauma care must be the maintenance of life, but there has been increasing emphasis, particularly since the early 1960s on what have more recently become known as quality of life issues.

> As the science of medicine has advanced, so the art of medicine appears to have declined.
>
> (Fallowfield, 1990)

While formal definition of quality of life remains nebulous, a number of concepts appear generally accepted, since the 1940s as indicative of a 'good life'. Initially these centred around materialistic attainment, then the Commission on National Goals established by President Eisenhower in 1960 extended the concept to include education, health and welfare, economic and industrial growth and 'the defense of the free world'. Since the 1970s greater pressure has been exerted by patients on health services, with greater emphasis placed on examining quality of life during illness and treatment. Indeed this reflects earlier established views held in the constitution of the World Health Organization (WHO, 1947), which stresses health as

> physical, mental and social well-being and not merely the absence of disease or infirmity.
>
> (WHO, 1947)

Quality of life was shown in Chapter 3 to be generally described as a quantifiable estimation of happiness or satisfaction with those aspects of life which are important to the specific individual, with quality synonymous with satisfaction, and overall life satisfaction as the embodiment of how well personal goals match with personal achievement. The objective and subjective measures associated with quality of life following spinal cord injury are well summarized by Ditunno (1997) and are highlighted below:

- *Objective measures*   Impairment, disability, handicap, medical complication, survival, health status.
- *Subjective measures*   Personal relationships, living arrangements, social life, recreation, finance, sex life, employment, overall satisfaction with life.

Society is at long last moving towards recognizing, if not yet accepting, that the problems experienced by those with disability are not simply due to intrapersonal difficulty or conflict, but are often the consequences of a disabling environment (Swain *et al.*, 1994).

Disability Politics

However, there remains a gulf between the injured person's perceptions of what constitutes disability and society's acceptance of the complications that impairment to, in this case, the spinal cord presents. Attributing responsibility for inability to live in a community should not simply be placed with the person who has the disability. Indeed the whole concept of disability needs to be viewed in a wider social and political framework, rather than relating purely to a medical framework. Tennant (1997), in a critical review of models of disability, stresses the need for wider debate when defining disability

> We should ensure that debate is open to all groups and includes all the issues. Increasing emphasis must be given to the enfranchisement of all disabled people involved in the health and social care process ... professionals should not be afraid to recognize the policy relevance of, and political nature of, disability, even if these matters are largely outside their sphere of influence.
>
> (Tennant, 1997: 478-479)

That people with disabilities are themselves increasingly influencing the views of society in general, and through directing how research in the area is conducted, is important (Oliver, 1990). Such work attempts to develop a more balanced view of need, away from research that attempts to alleviate or cure the effects of an impairment (positivism), to include experiences and feelings of those who have experienced the effects of disability (social constructionism). Extending such approaches further to include the role of environments (as would occur in functional analysis) begins to develop a dynamic framework within which society and communities play a significant part in making disability more extensive than the causal condition should present.

Johnston (1996) further questioned the validity of the World Health Organization (WHO) International Classification of Impairments, Disabilities and Handicaps (ICIDH) and suggested that inclusion of the theory of planned behaviour allowed more appropriate examination of the effects of impairment on attitudinal development, and perceived control over the behaviours which characterize disability.

You prepare yourself for the fact that the house will be difficult to get around. You even get used to the fact that a lot of people who called themselves your mates don't hang around once you get home. But the issue which annoys me most is that no matter where I go I'm constantly reminded that I'm 'different'. Trains don't have special facilities for my chair, people don't like me coming into their night clubs because I'm a fire risk, the local art gallery can only be reached up a flight of stairs. If I lived in America I'd join a rights movement; in Britain we're too reserved, we don't like to make a fuss. It's about time politicians in Britain were shaken out of their complacency and started to wake up to the fact that [we] vote and pay taxes and there comes a point at which every single person, without exception, says enough is enough. (Male, 32, C5 sensory incomplete tetraplegia)

It is indeed an indictment of the prevailing legal system in the United Kingdom that until 1995 it was perfectly lawful to discriminate against someone on the grounds that they have a disability. Changes proposed to this system were agreed by the government at that time. This act conferred two new rights upon people with disabilities: a right not to be discriminated against when applying for or when already in employment, and a right to access to services facilities and goods.

The Disability Discrimination Act (DDA) entered the statute books in 1995 with the remit of addressing employment rights for those with a wide range of disabilities. However, even before the DDA came into force, concerns were raised regarding its applicability. The definition of disability applied in the drafting was considered by many disabled groups as too complex and vague, and there was concern over how the new legislation might be fairly applied. In concluding her critique of the proposals Lawson (1995) states some important associated gains of well drafted legislation:

> It is clear from this brief summary of the Bill that the controversy that surrounded its introduction will also characterize its passage through Parliament . . . For the moment it appears that disabled people must be satisfied with the Government's measure or nothing. In one sense, this Bill may be worse than nothing in that it may have the effect of losing support for a more radical and comprehensive measure in the future.
>
> It is probably the feared costs of wider protection which have dictated the shape of the Bill. However . . . it should be remembered that disability legislation is not a measure for the benefit of some minority group which it has become politically correct to support. The Bill is something which could benefit us all . . . With an aging population, an increasing proportion will experience sensory impairments and mobility difficulties. As time proceeds and more buildings and services become accessible to disabled people, the benefits will be felt by a considerably larger part of the population.
>
> (Lawson, 1995: 152-153)

Since the DDA entered the statute books, a number of areas it addresses remain contentious:

1. The DDA allows for 'justifiable discrimination' provided employers make 'reasonable adjustment' to the working environment. Both issues are open to interpretation and such lack of clarity may well have dissuaded a number of people with disabilities from making a claim under the new legislation. However, government figures show that over 5,000 cases have been lodged since the DDA came into effect and that the rate of application is currently over 250 per month.

2. The onus is placed on the individual with the disability to prove they are disabled. The functional definitions applied within the DDA reinforce the negative aspects of the individual's impairment and can make the process of application extremely negative and distressing.

The establishment of a Disability Rights Commission has been proposed by the current government to support individuals in taking their cases forward. They have also established a Disability Rights Taskforce to address the areas of contention within the DDA. This group is currently addressing the issues of applicability under the act and whether education provision may be included in subsequent amendments to ensure equitability of access for those in all forms of education.

The DDA is seen by all interested groups as requiring radical revision. Although a number of claims for discrimination have been settled, with the issues regarding goods and services only to be enacted in October 1999, and equitability of access not due for implementation until 2004, it is too soon to comment on whether the DDA may yet have a fundamental impact on the lives of people with disabilities.

Garber *et al.* (1988) similarly suggest that the picture in the USA is not as supportive as people with disabilities in the UK might suppose. They indicate that 25–50 per cent of those with high tetraplegia are unable to obtain appropriate electric wheelchair allocation because of federal and insurance company funding restrictions. The delay in wheelchair allocation is also marked in the UK, and as funding restrictions have begun to bite here also, therapy staff are frequently faced with confronting service suppliers as advocates for the people they treat. The inclusion of such skills in professional qualification training is generally lacking, and academic course organizers continue to ignore it at their peril. The challenge for psychosocial research in the 21st century is summarized by Roberta Trieschmann (1992):

Without a doubt, survival with spinal cord injury depends on the acquisition of impeccable self care skills and the ability to tune into body function to anticipate trouble before it becomes a problem. But in order to live, not only survive, the person needs to face a society which frequently sends the message that you do not belong (through inaccessible environments), that you are different (through anxiety or avoidance by non-disabled people in social environments), and that you are now a second class citizen (through a programme of financial disincentives which penalise attempts to become productive and financially self-sufficient). How do we teach people to cope with these barriers? This is the focus for research.

(Trieschmann, 1992: 59)

While it is important to look for answers outside the immediacy of the study of spinal cord injury, it is important also to address the latent and explicit discrimination which exists within. This is particularly pertinent for women following spinal cord injury. The failure to adequately address sexual function was discussed in Chapter 5, but women with spinal cord injury are continually disenfranchised by both health care services, where males continue to dominate the medical profession, and society itself. As Trieschmann further notes:

Women with SCI fight the dual minority status of being not only a woman but also disabled. Often she is disenfranchised from long term relationships because a man's status is often judged by the physical perfection of his mate. Yet we know little about the coping ability of women with severe disability because they are infrequently the subject of research. Clinical observation reveals that women, in contrast to their frail and helpless image, are exceedingly strong and have significant resources to cope despite the lack of interpersonal support which many men have.

(Trieschmann, 1992: 60)

It is interesting to note that in Sweden, where political and social provision is more in harmony with the needs of those with disabilities, there was no difference in perceived quality of life between specific spinal cord lesion and control groups (Siosteen *et al.*, 1990). While Trieschmann's view holds true, it must be extended not only to include concerted attempts to enable people to cope with the situation which prevails, but also to advocate positive change at individual, family and societal levels. Removing the barriers to total equality for people with disability remains the greatest challenge as time passes into the new millennium.

Summary

The past 50 years have seen considerable developments in reducing death rates and complications for those with spinal cord injury. It may be considered, with limited exceptions, that the life expectancy for those with spinal cord injury is now comparable to the able bodied population. Electrically induced standing, and even assisted walking, is becoming more established, albeit presently for a selected group of people. Similarly, the next 10 years are likely to show even greater understanding of the processes of neurotransmission and methods to develop spinal regeneration.

However there remains the need to consider, with comparable personal and financial investment, the psychosocial needs of those toward whom developments are made. As societies become technically more advanced and the pace of life increases, the needs of the individual and the family often become submerged by the needs of the common ground. Within the global categorizations of spinal trauma there are implications for the remaining ability and resultant disability which are unique to each individual person. Spinal injury is not, therefore, simply another trauma or condition to which medical advance alone holds the answers. Patients and clinicians alike have often commented that 'about 80 per cent of coping with disability is what goes on in the person's head'. If clinicians and politicians alike remember the uniqueness of each spinal trauma and the simple truth that there but for the grace of whatever god they hold dear goes each of us, then services will continue to improve. The commercialization of western health care and the increasing competitiveness of service and research funding serves only to fragment constructive efforts towards co-operation and pooling of developments. Despite this codicil the experience of the author in working with those with spinal cord injury highlighted the positive approach to loss shown by the vast majority of patients and families, in the face of often seemingly insurmountable disadvantage.

Able bodied people have frequently commented that they wouldn't cope if they were faced with the same situation. It would be wrong to understate the implications of spinal cord injury. Considerable alteration in lifestyle does occur. Such a trauma draws on all the reserves of everyone involved. There are times when each person will consider they have had enough. However, the final message which must be given is one of hope:

When I got down to casualty I expected the worst. I was relieved when they said he wasn't dead. I was more relieved when I was told he didn't have a brain injury. When they told me he was going to Southport to get his back fixed I was ecstatic. When I got to Southport and I realized I hadn't been given the full picture about his back and that he'd need a wheelchair for the rest of his life I cried and cried. I felt I'd never cope; that he'd never accept the wheelchair. It was like I had been cheated all over again. But as the months progressed and I saw the progress he was making ... what he could do ... that despite his injuries he wasn't helpless, it became a bit easier. It was like three steps forward and two back and even now, when things get rough, and I feel like throttling him, I think back to what I might have lost and it makes it that bit easier to cope with. Of course I wish he was as he was before the accident but, while we both continue to get something out of life, who are we to complain. Our life was turned upside down by the accident and it's no longer life as we knew it, but it's our life, we've adapted to it. We tolerate the changes and enjoy it despite everything, and as far as we are concerned all in all it's a bloody good life! Spinal injury isn't something you would wish on your worst enemy, but it occurred so we get on with it. It's not the end of the world I thought it was at the start. (Wife of male, 34, C6 complete tetraplegia)

Further Reading

Fawcett, J.W. (1998). Spinal cord repair: from experimental models to human application. *Spinal Cord, 36*, 811–817.
State of the art review outlining where research is likely to lead in the next few years. Note, the emphasis in this area is on improvement in function, not full restoration of pre-injury ability.

Trieschmann, R.B. (1992). Psychosocial research in spinal cord injuries: the state of the art. *Paraplegia, 30*, 58–60.
Reviews applications of current learning theory models to spinal cord injury and suggestions for research in the future.

Oliver, M. (1990). *The Politics of Disablement*. Basingstoke: Macmillan.
Excellent review of the limitations of medical model of disability and development of the social model of disability.

Swain, J., Finkelstein, V., French, S. and Oliver, M. (Eds) (1994). *Disabling Barriers – Enabling Environments*. London: Sage Publications.
Written in the main by those with disabilities and emphasizes the role disabled people themselves have adopted in raising awareness of disability issues in society.

Glossary

Adrenergic Adrenalin producing.

Afferent Nerves which carry sensory impulses to the CNS.

Autonomic Dysreflexia Exaggerated sympathetic response to extrinsic stimulus below the level of lesion.

Axon The part of the neurone which conducts impulses away from the cell body.

Brown sequard syndrome Results when one side of the spinal cord is damaged, such as due to a knife assault. Below the level of injury there is motor paralysis and loss of proprioception on the ipsilateral side and loss of pain, temperature and touch on the contralateral side.

Catheter A (usually) silicon tube which drains or delivers fluid to a range of body organs.

Cauda equina The portion of the spinal cord below L1. Injury involves mainly peripheral nerves resulting in variable pattern of sensory and motor loss.

Central cord injury Where injury is more to the centre than the periphery of the spinal cord, causing greater paralysis and loss in upper extremities as these nerve tracts are more centrally located. Occurs more frequently in older patients as arthritic changes often cause narrowing of spinal canal and greater opportunity for transmission of forces centrally.

Central nervous system (CNS) Central nervous system; the brain and spinal cord.

Cerebro-spinal fluid (CSF) Clear fluid formed by filtration of blood plasma in the ventricles of the brain from where it flows into the subarachnoid spaces and circulates over the brain and spinal cord (and within the cord to the conus medullaris), acting as a protective, shock absorbing fluid around these structures.

Complete injury Total paralysis and loss of sensation below the level of injury.

Compressional fracture Downward force on the head or through transferred shock of landing on base of spine often results in burst fracture to vertebrae.

Contralateral The opposite side.

Contusion An injury to any part of the body, where the skin remains intact.

Conus meudularis The lower end of the spinal cord to L1.

Demyelination Compromise of the outer covering of the spinal cord.

Dendrite Part of the neurone that conducts impulses towards the cell body.

Dermatome An area of skin innervated by sensory axons from one spinal root.

Detrusor The smooth muscle of the bladder.

Efferent Nerves that carry motor impulses from the CNS to the muscles.

Erythema A reddened area on the skin surface where there is no break to the skin.

Fibrosis Thickening of tissue, often due to repeated trauma to the same area.

Flaccid Muscle contractions (movements) are not present.

Flexion injury Where the head is forced forwards in trauma; can cause a wedge fracture to the vertebrae and/or ligamentous damage.

Ganglia A tissue which contains large numbers of nerve-cell bodies located outside the spinal cord.

Hydrohypotonic environment A darkened suspension tank designed to mimic the effects of sensory deprivation.

Hydronephrosis Dilation of the kidney due to a range of medical complications.

Hyperaesthesia Abnormally increased sensation

Hyperextension injury Where the head is forced backwards, often resulting in damage to spinous process, pedicles or intervertebral discs.

Hyperreflexic Muscles which are in spasm or over-contracted.

Hypoaesthesia Reduction of sensation.

Hypo/hyper-thermia Condition of critically lowered/raised temperature which results when the body is unable to maintain a stable temperature, often due to damage to the autonomic nervous system.

Incidence The frequency of occurrence (usually reported annually) of a specific condition.

Incomplete spinal trauma Where there is some motor and/or sensory sparing below the level of injury to the spinal cord.

Ipsilateral On the same side.

Laminectomy A surgical procedure used to remove part of the vertebrae to gain access to the spinal cord.

Lateral flexion injury Where the head is forced forwards and to the side, injury can often result in wedge vertebral fracture.

Lower motor neurone (LMN) Originates within the spinal cord and receives impulses from UMNs. The LMNs travel outside the CNS to provide motor impulses to specific muscle groups and receive sensory information from the body back to the UMN in the spinal cord.

LMN injury Commonly identified when occurs at or below T12. Patient shows flaccid paralysis of the lower limbs and atonic bowel and bladder. Men with complete LMN below this level will be unable to obtain reflex erections.

Mortality Death rate associated with a specific condition.

Morbidity Frequency and nature of complications associated with a specific condition.

Myotome A group of muscle fibres innervated by a single spinal segment.

Neurogenic Originating within the nervous tissues.

Neurone Basic functional and anatomical unit within the CNS.

Neuronal hyperactivity Over-excitation of nerve fibres.

Neuropathic pain Pain caused by damage to nerve fibres either outside (peripheral) or within (central) the spinal cord.

Neuropathy Literally, nerve death.

Orthosis External support.

Paraparesis Weakness of the lower limbs and extremities.

Parasympathetic nervous system Fibres originate mainly in the 10th cranial (vagus) nerve and supply the heart, lungs and most organs in the abdomen. Fibres which originate in the sacral segments of the spinal cord supply the bladder and distal parts of the colon. During rest is more dominant for digestion and elimination purposes.

Pedicle Bony extension of vertebral body allowing rotation within a specific range and protection of the spinal cord.

Perceptual deprivation Reduction in sensory information received by any or all sensory organs.

Postural hypotension Uncontrolled reduction in blood pressure due to too rapid movement to upright posture.

Prevalence The total number of cases.

Priapism Persistent erection due to abnormal cause.

Proprioception Positional awareness.

Psychogenic response Actions mediated by conscious thought.

Reflex arc Path travelled by an impulse from a receptor to an effector organ not under volitional control (e.g. knee jerk in response to tap with patella hammer).

Reflux Backflow of urine from the bladder, through the ureters to kidneys.

Rotational injury Twisting of the spine about the long axis which often produces vertebral fracture and ligamentous damage.

Sensory deprivation Total ablation of sensory input to any or all sensory organs.

Spasm Involuntary muscle contraction.

Sphincter Small muscle with capacity to open or close a passage, such as occurs in controlling bowel and bladder outflow.

Spinal cord A complex extension of the brain in vertebrates controlling a number of bodily functions associated with control of organs to maintain homeostasis.

Spinal shock State caused by sudden cessation of efferent impulses which occurs immediately after spinal cord injury.

Spinous process Dorsal bony extension of vertebral body. Provides dorsal protection to the spinal cord.

Sympathetic nervous system Neurones which secrete norepinephrine/noradrenaline preparing the body to deal with stress. The fibres originate in the grey matter of the spinal cord. Controls the blood vessels and sweat glands throughout the body. Also causes autonomic cord reflexes or transmit sensory impulses to the brain via the ascending tracts.

Tetraparesis Weakness of all four limbs and extremities.

Trauma Injury to the body or organ system.

Upper motor neurone (UMN) Originates in the brain and is located within the spinal cord.

Umn lesion Occurs at or above T12 and produces spasticity of limbs below level of injury, increased muscle tone and spasticity of the bladder and bowel.

Urethra Communicating passage between bladder and perineum.

Ureter Communicating tube between the bladder and each kidney.

Organizations, Useful Addresses and Web Pages

Organizations

American Spinal Injuries Association (ASIA), 2020 Peachtree Road NW, Atlanta, Georgia 30309.

The Back-Up Trust, The Business Village, Broomhill Road, London, SW18 4JQ (Tel: 0181 875 1805; Fax: 0181 870 3619; email: back-up@dial.pipex.com).

International Medical Society of Paraplegia (IMSOP), National Spinal Injuries Centre, Stoke Mandeville Hospital, Aylesbury, Buckinghamshire, HP21 8AL.

International Spine Research Trust (ISRT), Nicholas House, River Front, Enfield, Middlesex, EN1 3TR.

National Spinal Cord Injury Association (NSCIA), 600 West Cummings Park, Suite 2000, Woburn, Massachusetts 01801.

Paralyzed Veterans of America, 801 18th Street North West, Washington DC 20006.

Spinal Injuries Association (SIA), Newpoint House, 76 St James's Lane, London, N10 3DF.

Specialist Spinal Injuries Centres in the United Kingdom

Hexham General Hospital, Hexham, NE46 1QJ (Tel: 01434 606161).

Musgrave Park Hospital, Belfast, BT9 7JB (Tel: 01232 669501).

Northern General Hospital, Sheffield, S5 7AU (Tel: 0114 2434343).

Our Lady of Lourdes Hospital, Dun Laoghaire, Dublin (Tel: + 35 35 285477).

Pinderfields General Hospital, Wakefield, WF1 4EE (Tel: 01924 201688).

Robert Jones and Agnes Hunt Orthopaedic Hospital, Oswestry, ST10 7AG (Tel: 01691 404000).

Salisbury District General Hospital, Salisbury, SP2 8BJ (Tel: 01722 336262).

Southern General Hospital, Glasgow, G51 4TF (Tel: 0141 2012555).

Southport District General Hospital, Southport, Merseyside, PR8 6PN (Tel: 01704 547471).

Stoke Mandeville Hospital, Aylesbury, HP21 8AL (Tel: 01296 315000).

Internet Addresses and Web Pages

http://www.spinalcord.org/ National Spinal Cord Injury Association
Provides links to a wide range of other resources. The correct email address is listed on the page.

http://www.noah.cuny.edu/illness/neuro/spinal.html
Ask Noah about: Spinal and Head Injuries
Provides links to a wide selection of links regarding spinal and head injuries.

http://www.cureparalysis.org
Up-to-date statistics on incidence and prevalence and some good pictures.

http://www.backup.org.uk The Back-Up Trust
Aims to increase motivation, inspiration and independence through outdoor, adventurous activities for those paralysed through spinal cord injury.

http://www.qbg.org Quadriplegia by gunfire
A site hosted and maintained by a C5 tetraplegic. Has a variety of links to other information and links to other spinally injured people.

http://glaxocentre.merseyside.org/sia.html
Spinal Injuries Association (SIA)
Provides links and information on various sources as well as a list of publications concerning a wide range of spinal injury related topics. The main SIA association site is at http://igweb.com/SIA/.

http://www.copernicus.win-uk.net/rehab.htm
As the name might suggest, lots of useful information and loads of links to other topics and information sites.

http://www.spinalcord.uab.edu
Spinal Cord Injury Information Network

http://www.asia-spinalinjury.org
American Spinal Injuries Association (ASIA)
Good reviews of news and happenings in the USA systems, and good search facilities.

http://www.ohsu.edu/cliniweb/C21/C21.866.html#C21.866.819
This is a library of information on all the physical aspects of spinal cord injury. Excellent.

http://www.nlm.nih.gov
The United States National Library of Medicine

References

Aaronson, N. (1988). Quality of life: What is it? How should it be measured? *Oncology, 2,* 5, 69–74.

Abramson, L.Y., Seligman, M.E.P. and Teasdale, J.D. (1978). Learned helplessness in humans: Critique and reformulation. *Journal of Abnormal Psychology.* *87,* 49–74.

Aguiler, D. and Mesgick, J. (1978). *Crisis Intervention: Theory and Methodology.* St Louis, MO: Mosby.

American Spinal Injuries Association (1992). *Standards for Neurological and Functional Classification of Spinal Cord Injury.* Chicago, IL: American Spinal Injuries Association.

Anderson, C.J. and Mulcahey, M.J. (1997). Menstruation and paediatric spinal cord injury. *Journal of Spinal Cord Medicine, 20,* 1, 56–59.

Bach, J.R. and Tilton, M.C. (1994). Life satisfaction and well-being measures in ventilator assisted individuals with traumatic tetraplegia. *Archives of Physical Medicine and Rehabilitation, 75,* 626–632.

Baker, E.R. and Cardenas, D.D. (1996). Pregnancy in spinal cord women. *Archives of Physical Medicine and Rehabilitation, 77,* 5, 501–507.

Bandura, A. (1969). *Principles of Behaviour Modification.* New York: Holt Rinehart & Winston.

Bandura, A. (1986). *Social Foundations of Thought and Action: A Social Cognitive Model.* Upper Saddle River, NJ: Prentice Hall.

Bandura, A., Taylor, C.B., Williams, S.L., Mefford, I.N., and Barchas, J.D. (1985). Catecholamine secretion as a function of perceived coping self-efficacy. *Journal of Consulting and Clinical Psychology, 53* 406–414.

Banja, J.D. (1990). Rehabilitation and empowerment. *Archives of Physical Medicine and Rehabilitation, 71,* 614–615.

Barbenel, J.C. and Paul, J.P. (1992). Bioengineering developments for paraplegic patients. *Paraplegia, 30,* 61–64.

Beck, A.T., Weissman, A., Lester, D. and Trexler, L. (1974). The measurement of pessimism: The Hopelessness Scale. *Journal of Consulting and Clinical Psychology, 42,* 861–865.

Becker, E.F. (1978). *Female Sexuality Following Spinal Cord Injury.* Bloomington, IL: Cheever Publishing.

Bennett, C.J., McCabe, M., Ayers, J.W.T., Moinipanah, R., Randolph, J.F., McGuire, E.J. and Seager, S.W.J. (1987). Electroejaculation of paraplegic males followed by pregnancies. *Fertility and Sterility, 48,* 1070–1073.

Berkman, P.L. (1971). Measurement of mental health in a general population survey. *American Journal of Epidemiology, 94,* 105–111.

Black, K., Sipski, M.L. and Strauss, S.S. (1998). Sexual satisfaction and sexual drive in spinal cord injured women. *Journal of Spinal Cord Medicine, 21,* 3, 240–244.

Bogle, J., Hudgins, G., Peters, L., Shaul, S. and Wysocki, J. (1980). *Manual for Service Providers.* Washington DC: Ebon Research Systems.

Bonica, J.J. (1991). Introduction: semantic, epidemiological and educational issues. In K.L. Casey (Ed.) *Pain and Central Nervous System Disease: The Central Pain Syndromes*. New York: Raven Press.

Boudurant, E.J. (1990). Acute spinal cord injury: a study using physical examination and MRI. *Spine, 15*, 161–168.

Brag, G.P. (1977). Reactive patterns in families of the severely disabled. *Rehabilitation Counselling Bulletin, 20*, 236–239.

Bregman, S. and Hadley, R.G. (1976) Sexual adjustment and feminine attractiveness among spinal cord injured women. *Archives of Physical Medicine and Rehabilitation, 57*, 215–227.

Buckelew, S.P., Frank, R.G., Elliott, T.R., Chaney, J. and Hewitt, J. (1991). Adjustment to spinal cord injury: Stage theory revisited. *Paraplegia, 29*, 125–130.

Burke, D.C. and Murray, D.D. (1975). *Handbook of Spinal Cord Medicine*. Basingstoke: Macmillan.

Campbell, A. (1976). Subjective measures of well-being. *American Psychologist, 31*, 117–124.

Carter, R.E. (1993). Experiences with ventilator dependent patients. *Paraplegia, 31*, 150–153.

Cassata, M. (1982). In M.R. DiMatteo and D.D. DiNicola (1982). *Achieving Patient Compliance: The Psychology of the Medical Practitioner's Role*. New York: Pergamon: p. 45.

Chapelle, P.A., Durand, J. and Lacert, P. (1992). Penile erection following complete spinal cord injury in man. *British Journal of Urology, 52*, 216–219.

Cheng, C.Y., Ho, K.W. and Leung, K.K. (1993). Multi-adjustable post-operative orthosis for congenital muscular torticollis. *Prosthetics and Orthotics International, 17*, 2, 115–119.

Christopherson, J. (1968). Role modifications of the disabled male. *American Journal of Nursing, 68*, 290–293.

Clement, V. and Schmidt, G. (1983). The outcome of couple therapy for sexual dysfunctions using three different formats. *Journal of Sexual and Marital Therapy, 9*, 1, 67–80.

Cohen, F. (1987). Measurement of coping. In S.V. Kasl and C.L. Cooper (Eds) *Stress and Health: Issues in Research Methodology*. New York: Wiley.

Cole, S.S. (1988). Women, sexuality and disability. *Women and Therapy, 7*, 277–294.

Cooper, A. (1969). Disorders of sexual potency in the male: a clinical and statistical study of some factors related to short term prognosis. *British Journal of Psychiatry, 115*, 709–719.

Crewe, N.M. (1991). Ageing and severe physical disability: patterns of change and implications for services. *International Disability Studies, 13*, 158–161.

Crewe, N.M. and Krause, J.S. (1988). Marital relationships and spinal cord injury. *Archives of Physical Medicine and Rehabilitation, 69*, 435–438.

Crewe, N.M. and Krause, J.S. (1992). Marital status and adjustment to spinal cord injury. *Journal of the American Paraplegia Society, 15*, 14–18.

Crossman, M.W. (1996). Sensory deprivation in spinal cord injury – an essay. *Paraplegia, 34*, 573–577.

Cushman, L. and Dijkers, M. (1990). Depressed mood in spinal cord injury patients: staff perceptions and patient reactions. *Archives of Physical Medicine and Rehabilitation, 71,* 191–196.

David, S. and Aguayo, A.J. (1981). Axonal elongation into peripheral nervous system bridges after central nervous system injury. *Science, 241,* 931–933.

Decker, S. Schultz, R. and Wood, D. (1989). Determinants of well being in primary care givers of spinal cord injured persons. *Rehabilitation Nursing, 14,* 1, 6–8.

Dell Fitting, M., Salisbury, S., Davies, N. and Mayclin, D.K. (1978). Self-concept and sexuality of spinal cord injured women. *Archives of Sexual Behaviour, 7,* 143–156.

Derogatis, L.R. and Melisaratos, N. (1983). The Brief Symptoms Inventory: an introductory report. *Psychological Medicine, 13,* 595–605.

Derry, F.A., Dinsmore, W.W., Fraser, M., Gardner, B.P., Glass, C.A., Maytom, M. and Smith, M.D. (1998). Efficacy and safety of oral sildenafil (Viagra) in men with erectile dysfunction caused by spinal cord injury. *Neurology, 51,* 629–1633.

DeVivo, M.J., Black, K.J., Richards, J.S. and Stover, S.L. (1991). Suicide following spinal cord injury. *Paraplegia, 29,* 9, 620–627.

DeVivo, M.J. and Ivie, C.S. (1995). Life expectancy of ventilator-dependent persons with spinal cord injuries. *Chest, 108,* 1, 226–232.

Ditunno, J.F. (1997). Functional outcomes in spinal cord injury: quality care versus cost containment. *Journal of Spinal Cord Medicine, 20,* 1, 1–7.

Doll, B. and Michael, T. (1994). Current Status of orthotic management of children with meningomyelocele. *Z. Orthop. Ihre. Grenzgeb.* (Germany), *123,* 3, 201–206.

Donovan, W.H., Carter, R.E., Bedbrook, G., Young, J.S. and Griffiths, E.R. (1984). Incidence of medical complications in spinal cord injury: patients in specialized compared with non-specialized centres. *Paraplegia, 22,* 282–290.

Ducharme, S.H. and Freed, M.M. (1980). The role of self destruction in spinal cord injury mortality. *Spinal Cord Injury Digest, 2,* 4, 29–38.

Eide, P.K. (1998). Pathophysiological mechanisms of central neuropathic pain after spinal cord injury. *Spinal Cord, 36,* 9, 601–612.

Elliott, T.R. and Frank, R.G. (1996). Depression following spinal cord injury. *Archives of Physical Medicine and Rehabilitation, 77,* 816–823.

Epstein, L.H. and Cuss, P.A. (1982). A behavioural medicine perspective on adherence to long-term medical regimens. *Journal of Consulting and Clinical Psychology, 50,* 950–971.

Fallowfield, L. (1990). *The Quality of Life: The Missing Measurement in Health Care.* London: Souvenir Press.

Fallowfield, L.J., Baum, M. and Maguire, G.P. (1986). Effects of breast conservation on psychological morbidity associated with diagnosis and treatment of early breast cancer. *British Medical Journal, 293,* 1331–1334.

Fawcett, J.W. (1998). Spinal cord repair: from experimental models to human application. *Spinal Cord, 36,* 811–817.

Ferrans, C.E. (1990). Quality of life: conceptual issues. *Seminars in Oncology Nursing* 248–254.

Ferrans, C.E. and Powers, M.J. (1986). Quality of Life Index: development and psychometric properties. *Advances in Nursing Science, 8*, 1, 15–24.

Ferrans, C.E. and Powers, M.J. (1992). Psychometric assessment of the Quality of Life. *Index of Research Nursing and Health, 15*, 29–38.

Ford, A.B. and Orifier, A.P. (1967). Sexual behaviour and the chronically ill patient. *Medical Aspects of Human Sexuality, 10*, 51–61.

Fordyce, W.E. (1976). *Behavioural Methods for Chronic Pain and Illness.* St Louis, MO: Mosby.

Frankel, H.L., Hancock, D.O. and Hyslop, G. (1969). The value of postural reduction in the initial management of closed injuries of the spine with paraplegia and tetraplegia. *International Journal of Paraplegia, 7*, 1, 179–192.

Fraser, M.H. and Holmes, T. (1990). The Southport professional rehabilitation programme. *2nd International Meeting of Robotics and Handicap*, 218.

Frederico, D.J. and Renshaw, T.S. (1990). Results of treatment of idiopathic scoliosis with the Charleston bending orthosis, *Spine, 15* 9, 886–887.

Fuhrer, M.J., Carter, R.E., Donovan, W.H. *et al.* (1987). Postdischarge outcomes for ventilator-dependent quadriplegics. *Archives of Physical Medicine and Rehabilitation, 68*, 353–356.

Garber, S.L., Letham, P. and Gregorio, T.L. (1988). *Specialized Occupational Therapy for Persons with High Level Quadriplegia.* Houston, TX: Institute for Rehabilitation Research.

Gardner, B.P., Theocleous, F., Watt, J.W.H. and Krishnan, K.R. (1985). Ventilation or dignified death for patients with high tetraplegia. *British Medical Journal, 291*, 1620–1622.

George, L. and Bearon, L. (1980). *Quality of Life in Older Persons.* New York: Human Sciences Press.

Glass, C.A. (1993). The impact of home based ventilation on family life. *International Journal of Paraplegia, 31*, 93–101.

Glass, C.A. (1992). Applying functional analysis to psychological rehabilitation following spinal cord injury. *Journal of the American Paraplegia Society, 15*, 187–193.

Glass, C.A., Fielding, D.M., Evans, C.M. and Ashcroft, J.B. (1987). Factors related to sexual functioning in male patients undergoing haemodialysis and after kidney transplants. *Archives of Sexual Behaviour, 16* 3, 189–207.

Glass, C.A., Krishnan, K.R., Fraser, M.H., Jones, J. and Holmes, T. (1991a). The Southport Project: A Collaborative Venture in Retraining the Profoundly Disabled Due to Spinal Cord Injury; Psychological Perspectives. *Proceedings of the 5th European Health Society Conference*, Lausanne.

Glass, C.A., Krishnan, K.R. and Bingley, J.D. (1991b). Spinal injury rehabilitation: do staff and patients agree on what they are talking about? *Paraplegia, 29*, 343–349.

Glass, C.A., Watt, J.W.H., Krishnan, K.R., Bingley, J.D. and Orritt, C.M. (1996). A comparison of quality of life following spinal cord injury for those who require permanent home ventilation (PHV) and those who had received phrenic nerve implants (PNI). *European Journal of Neurology, 3*, 2, 32–33.

Glass, C.A., Charlifue, S.W., Dutton, J., Jackson, H.F. and Orritt, C. (1997). Who gives a better estimation of social adjustment following spinal trauma – patient or spouse? 1: a statistical justification. *Spinal Cord, 35*, 320–325.

Glass, C.A., Charlifue, S.W., Dutton, J., Jackson, H.F. and Orritt, C. (1997a). Who gives a better estimation of social adjustment following spinal trauma – patient or spouse? 2: Effects of compensation on adjustment. *Spinal Cord, 35*, 349–357.

Glass, C.A., Derry, F., Dinsmore, W.W., Fraser, M., Gardner, B., Maytom, M., Orr, M., Osterloh, I. and Smith, M. (1997b). Sildenafil: an oral treatment for men with erectile dysfunction caused by traumatic spinal cord injury – a double blind, placebo controlled, two way crossover study using Rigiscan. *Journal of Spinal Cord Medicine, 20*, 1, 145.

Glen, W.L. and Phelps, M.L. (1985). Diaphragm pacing by electrode stimulation of the phrenic nerve. *Neurosurgery, 17*, 974–980.

Granger, C.V. (1985). Outcome of comprehensive medical rehabilitation: an analysis based upon the impairment, disability, and handicap model. *International Rehabilitation Medicine, 7*, 45–50.

Granger, C.V., Albrecht, G.L. and Hamilton, B.B. (1979). Outcome of comprehensive medical rehabilitation: measurement by PULSES profile and Barthel Index. *Archives of Physical Medicine and Rehabilitation, 60*, 145–154.

Granger, C.V., Cotter, A.C., Hamilton, B.B., Fiedler, R.C. and Hens, M.M. (1990). Functional assessment scales: a study of persons with multiple sclerosis. *Archives of Physical Medicine and Rehabilitation, 71*, 870–875.

Gresham, G.E., Labi, M., Dittmar, S., Hicks, J., Joyce, S. and Phillips Stehik, M. (1986). The quadriplegic index of function (QIF): sensitivity and reliability demonstrated in a study of 30 quadriplegic patients. *Paraplegia, 24*, 38–44.

Harris, P., Patel, S., Greer, W. and Naughton, M.C. (1973). Psychological and social reactions to acute spinal paralysis. *Paraplegia, 11*, 132–136.

Harrison, J., Glass, C.A., Owens, R.G. and Soni, B.M. (1995). Sexual functioning in women following spinal cord injury. *International Journal of Paraplegia, 33*, 687–692.

Hawton, K. (1987). Assessment of suicide risk. *British Journal of Psychiatry, 150*, 145–153.

Haynes, R.B. (1982). Improving patient compliance: an empirical review. In R.B. Stuart (Ed.) *Adherence, Compliance, and Generalization in Behavioural Medicine*. New York: Bruner Mazel.

Heinemann, A.W., Yarkony, G.M., Roth, E.J., Lovell, L., Hamilton, B., Ginsburg, K., Brown, J.T. and Meyer, P.R. (1989). Functional outcome following spinal cord injury: a comparison of specialized spinal cord centre vs general hospital short term care. *Archives of Neurology, 46*, 1098–1102.

Higgins, G.E. (1979). Sexual response in spinal cord injured adults: a review of the literature. *Archives of Sexual Behaviour, 8*, 173–196.

Hirsch, S.R., Walsh, C. and Draper, R. (1982). Parasuicide: a review of treatment interventions. *Journal of Affective Disorders, 4*, 299–311.

Hoad, A.D., Oliver, M.J. and Silver, J.R. (1990). *The experience of spinal cord injury for other family members*. London: Thames Polytechnic Publications.

Hogbin, B.J. and Fallowfield, L.J. (1989). Getting it taped: the 'bad news' consultation in a general surgical outpatients department. *British Journal of Hospital Medicine, 41*, 330–333.

Hohman, G.W. (1966). Some effects of spinal cord lesions on experienced emotional feelings. *Psychophysiology. 3*, 2, 143–156.

Holmes, D.M. (1986). The person and diabetes in social context. *Diabetes Care, 9*, 194–206.

Hooper, M. (1994a). *Sexuality and Spinal Cord Injury: Heterosexual Men.* London: Spinal Injuries Association.

Hooper, M. (1994b). *Sexuality and Spinal Cord Injury: Heterosexual Women.* London: Spinal Injuries Association.

Hooper, M. and Regard (1994a). *Sexuality and Spinal Cord Injury: Gay Men.* London: Spinal Injuries Association.

Hooper M and Regard (1994b). *Sexuality and Spinal Cord Injury: Lesbians.* London: Spinal Injuries Association.

Horvat, J.C. (1992). Neural transplants in spinal cord injury. *Paraplegia, 30*, 23–26.

Human Fertilization and Embryology Act (1990). *Code of Practice.* London: HFEA.

Hunter, J. (1988). *Bridging the Gap: Case Management and Advocacy for People with Physical Disabilities.* London: King Edwards Fund for London.

Jackson, H.F., Glass, C.A. and Hope, S. (1987). A functional analysis of recidivistic arson. *British Journal of Clinical Psychology, 26*, 175–185.

Jackson, H.F., Hopewell, C.A., Glass, C.A., Ghadiali, E. and Warberg, R. (1992). The Katz adjustment scale: modification for use with victims of brain and spinal injury. *Brain Injury, 6*, 2, 109–127.

Jehu, D. (1979). *Sexual Dysfunction: A Behavioural Approach to Causation, Assessment and Treatment.* Wiley: New York.

Johnston, M. (1996). Models of disability. *The Psychologist, 9*, 5, 205–210.

Johnston, M., Marteau, T., Partridge, C. and Gilbert, P. (1990). Changes in patient perceptions of chronic disease and disability with time and experience. In L.R. Schmidt, P. Schwenkmezger, J. Weinman and S. Maes (Eds) *Theoretical and Applied Aspects of Health Psychology.* Churchill: Harwood Academic Publishers.

Judd, F.K. and Brown, D.J. (1992). Suicide following traumatic spinal cord injury. *Paraplegia 30*, 173–177.

Junemann, K.P., Leu, T.F., Fournier Jr., G.R. and Tanegho, E.A. (1991). Review of therapy: pharmacology surgery methods in clinical urodynamics. *Dantec,* 24–27.

Kakulas, B.A. (1993). The applied neurobiology of human spinal cord injury: a review. Cited in P. Harris (1992). Spinal cord injuries in the 21st century. *Paraplegia, 30*, 31–34.

Katchadourian, H.A. (1990) *The Biological Aspects of Human Sexuality.* 4th ed. New York: Holt, Rinehart & Winston.

Katz, M.M. and Lyerley, S.B. (1963). Methods for measuring adjustment and social behaviour in the community: rationale, description, discriminative validity and scale development. *Psychological Reports, 13*, 503–535.

Keith, M.W., Hunter-Peckam, P., Thrope, G.B. (1989). Implantable functional neuromuscular stimulator in the tetraplegic hand. *Journal of Hand Surgery, 14*, 524–530.

Kennedy, P., Fisher, K. and Pearson, E. (1988). Ecological evaluation of a rehabilitative environment for spinal cord injured people. *British Journal of Clinical Psychology, 27*, 239–246.

Kennedy, P., Walker, L. and White, D. (1991). Ecological evaluation of goal planning and advocacy in a rehabilitative environment for spinal cord injured people. *Paraplegia. 29*, 197–202.

Kilgore, K.L., Hunter-Peckham, P. and Keith, M.W. (1995). An implanted upper extremity neuroprosthesis: a 20 patient follow-up. *Journal of Spinal Cord Medicine, 18*, 2, 147.

Kilgore, K.L., Hunter-Peckham, P. and Keith, M.W. (1997). An implanted upper extremity neuroprosthesis: a five patient follow-up. *Journal of Bone and Joint Surgery, 79*, 4, 533–541.

Kings Fund (1991). *Counselling for Regulated Infertility Treatments*. London: The Kings Fund.

Kitzinger, S. (1983). *Women's Experience of Sex*. New York: G.P. Puttnam and Sons.

Komisaruk, B.R. and Whipple, B. (1994). Complete spinal cord injury does not block perceptual responses to vaginal or cervical self-stimulation in women. *Society for Neuroscience Abstracts, 20*, 961.

Krause, J. (1990). The relationship of productivity to adjustment following spinal cord injury. *Rehabilitation Counselling Bulletin. 33*, 188–199.

Krause, J.S. and Crewe, N.M. (1991). Chronological age, time since injury, and time of measurement: effect on adjustment after spinal cord injury. *Archives of Physical Medicine and Rehabilitation, 72*, 91–100.

Kreuter, M., Sullivan, M. and Siosteen, A. (1994). Sexual adjustment after spinal cord injury focusing on partner experiences. *Paraplegia, 32*, 225–235.

Kreuter, M., Sullivan, M. and Siosteen, A. (1994). Sexual adjustment after spinal cord injury: comparison of partner experiences in pre- and post-injury relationships. *Paraplegia, 32*, 759–770.

Kreuter, M., Sullivan, M. and Siosteen, A. (1996). Sexual adjustment and quality of relationships in spinal paraplegia: a controlled study. *Archives of Physical Medicine and Rehabilitation, 77*, 541–548.

Krishnan, K.R. (1993). Recommendations concerning the costing and management for patients requiring domiciliary ventilation. *Paraplegia, 31*, 276–279.

Krishnan, K.R. (1994). Litigation after catastrophic injury: need for a change in trend. *Personal Injury Law and Medical Review, 1*, 342–352.

Krishnan, K.R., Fraser, M.H., Glass, C.A. and Whalley, T. (1991). Measuring rehabilitation outcomes in a spinal injuries centre. A programme to assess progress and quality. *Journal of the American Paraplegia Society, 14*, 2, 85.

Krishnan, K.R., Glass, C.A., Turner, S.M., Watt, J.W.H. and Fraser, M.H. (1992). Perceptual deprivation in the acute phase of spinal injury rehabilitation. *Journal of the American Paraplegia Society, 15*, 2, 60–65.

Kubler-Ross, E. (1969). *On Death and Dying*. New York: Macmillan.

Lasfargues, J.E., Custis, D., Morrone, F., Carswell, J. and Nguyen, T. (1995). A model for estimating spinal cord injury prevalence in the United States. *Paraplegia, 33*, 62–68.

Lawson J. (1995). Disability discrimination. The Disability Discrimination Act 1995. *Personal Injury, 3*, 140–155.

Lazarus, R.S. and Folkman, S. (1984). Coping and adaptation. In W. Gentry (Ed.) *Handbook of Behavioural Medicine.* London: Guilford.

Levenson, H. (1973). Activism and powerful others: distinctions within the concept of internal–external locus of control. *Journal of Personality Assessment. 38*, 377–383.

Levy, N.B. (1974). *Living or Dying: Adaptation To Haemodialysis.* Springfield, IL: Charles C. Thomas.

Ley, P. (1982). Satisfaction, compliance and communication. *British Journal of Clinical Psychology, 21*, 241–254.

Lyles, M. and Munday, J. (1992). Report on the evaluation of the Vannini–Rizzoli Stabilizing Limb Orthosis. *Journal of Rehabilitation Research Development, 29*, 2, 77–104.

MacLeod, A.K., Williams, J.M.G. and Linehan, G.I. (1992). New developments in the understanding and treatment of suicidal behaviour. *Behavioural Psychotherapy, 20*, 3,193–218.

MacLeod, G.M. and Macleod, L. (1996). Evaluation of client and staff satisfaction with a goal planning project implemented with people with spinal cord injuries. *Spinal Cord, 34*, 525–530.

Mahoney, F.I. and Barthel, D.W. (1965). Functional evaluation: the Barthel Index. *Mid State Medical Journal, 14*, 61–65.

Mariano, A.J. (1992) Chronic pain and spinal cord injury. *Clinical Journal of Pain, 8*, 87–92.

Marincek, C.R.T. (1988). Community based rehabilitation – the challenge and opportunity. *International Disability Studies, 10*, 87–88.

Marino, R.J., Huang, M., Knight, P., Herbison, G.J., Ditunno, J.F. and Segal, M. (1993). Assessing selfcare status in quadriplegia: comparison of the Quadriplegic Index of Function (QIF) and the Functional Independence Measure (FIM). *Paraplegia, 31*, 225–233.

Maris, R.W. (1981). *Pathways to Suicide.* London: John Hopkins Press.

Marrett, S., Evans, A.C. and Collins, I. (1988). Three dimensional MR–PET imaging in the human brain. *Radiology,* (Suppl.), 169–369.

Martin, J., Meltzer, H. and Elliot, D. (1988). The prevalence of disability among adults. *OPCS Survey of Disability in Great Britain, Report 1.* London: HMSO.

Mawson, A.R., Biundo, J.J., Neville, P., Linares, H.A., Winchester, Y. and Lopez, A. (1988). Risk factors for early occurring pressure ulcers following spinal cord injury. *American Journal of Physical Medicine and Rehabilitation, 40*, 123–127.

Maynard, F.M. and Muth, A.S. (1987). The choice to end life as a ventilator dependent quadriplegic. *Archives of Physical Medicine and Rehabilitation, 68*, 682–684.

Maytom, M.C., Derry, F.A., Dinsmore, W.W., Glass, C.A., Smith, M.D., Orr, M. and Osterloh, I.H. (1999). A two part pilot study of sildenafil (Viagra) in men with erectile dysfunction caused by spinal cord injury. *Spinal Cord, 37*, 110–116.

Moos, R.H. (1982). Coping with acute health crises. In T. Millon, C. Green and R. Meagher (Eds) *Handbook of Clinical Health Psychology*. New York: Plenum.

Morris, J. (Ed.) (1989). *Able Lives: Women's Experience of Paralysis*. London: Women's Press.

Mumenthaler, M. (1985) (translated by Appenzeller, O.). *Neurological Differential Diagnosis*. New York: Thieme-Stratton.

Nagler, B. (1950). Psychiatric aspects of cord injury. *American Journal of Psychiatry*, 107, 49–56.

Naylor, N.J. and Mulley, G.P. (1991). Surgical collars: a survey of their prescription and use. *British Journal of Rheumatology*, 30, 4, 282–284.

Neugarten, B.L., Havighurst, R.J. and Tobin, S.S. (1961). The measurement of life satisfaction. *Journal of Gerontology*, 16, 134–143.

Newman, S., Fitzpatrick, R., Lamb, R. and Shipley, M. (1990). An analysis of patterns of coping in rheumatoid arthritis. In L.R. Schmidt, P. Schwenkmezger, J. Weinman and S. Maes (Eds) *Theoretical and Applied Aspects of Health Psychology*. Churchill: Harwood Academic Publishers.

Norris Baker, C., Stephens, M. and Rinalta, D. (1981). Patient behaviour as a predictor of outcome in spinal cord injury. *Archives of Physiological and Medical Research*, 62, 602–608.

Nyquist, R. and Bors, E. (1967). Mortality and survival in traumatic myelopathy during nineteen years from 1946 to 1965. *Paraplegia*, 5, 22–48.

Office of Health Economics (1981). *Suicide and Deliberate Self Harm*. London.

Ohry, A., Gur, S. and Zeilig, G. (1989). Duplicate limb sensation in acute traumatic quadriplegia. *Paraplegia*, 27, 257–260.

Oliver, M. (1990). *The Politics of Disablement*. Basingstoke: Macmillan.

Oliver, M., Zarb, G. and Silver, J. (1988). *Walking into Darkness: The Experience of Spinal Cord Injury*. Basingstoke: Macmillan

Owens, R.G. and Ashcroft, J.B. (1982). Functional analysis in applied psychology. *British Journal of Clinical Psychology*, 21, 181–189.

Owens, R.G. and Naylor, F. (1989). *Living while Dying: What to Do and What to Say When You are, or Someone Close to You is Dying*. Northamptonshire: Thorsens Publishers.

Pachalski, A. and Pachalska, M.M. (1984). Programme of active education in the psycho-social Integration of paraplegics. *Paraplegia*, 22, 238–243.

Parrish, J.J. (1986). Parent compliance with medical and behavioural recommendations. In Krasnegor, N.A., Arasteh, J.D. and Cataldo, F. (Eds) *Child Health Behaviour: A Behavioural Paediatrics Perspective*. New York: Wiley.

Parsons, K.C. and Lamertse, D.P. (1991). Rehabilitation in spinal cord disorders: 1. Epidemiology, prevention and system of care of spinal cord disorders. *Archives of Physical Medicine and rehabilitation*, 72, 293–294.

Paykel, E.S., Prusoff, B.A. and Myers, J.K. (1975). Suicide attempts and recent life events. *Archives of General Psychiatry*, 32, 327–333.

Peck, C.L. and King, N.J. (1985). Compliance and the doctor–patient relationship. *Drugs*, 30, 78–84.

Perry, J.D. and Whipple, B. (1981). Pelvic muscle strength of female ejaculators: evidence in support of a new theory of orgasm. *Journal of Sex Research*, 17, 22–39.

Peyser, J.M., Edwards, K.R., and Poser, C.M. (1980). Psychological profiles in patients with multiple sclerosis. *Archives of Neurology, 37*, 437–440.

Phares, E.J. (1987). Locus of control. In R.L. Corsini (Ed.) *Concise Encyclopedia of Psychology*. New York: Wiley.

Purtillo, R.B. (1986). Ethical issues in treatment of chronic ventilator dependent patients. *Archives of Physical Medicine and Rehabilitation, 67*, 718–721.

Quellete, E.A. (1991). The rheumatoid hand: orthotics as preventative. *Seminars in Arthritis and Rheumatology, 21*, 2, 65–72.

Raisman, G. (1987). Genes and spine patients. *International Spinal Research Trust Newsletter 12*, 4–5.

Robinson, I. (1988). *Multiple Sclerosis*. London: Routledge.

Rollnick, S., Heather, N. and Bell, A. (1992). Negotiating behaviour change in medical settings: the development of brief motivational interviewing. *Journal of Mental Health, 1*, 25–37.

Rosenstock, I.M. (1985). Understanding and enhancing patient compliance with diabetic regimens. *Diabetic Care, 8*, 610–616.

Ryan, J. (1961). Dreams of paraplegics. *Archives of General Psychiatry, 5*, 94.

Sanders, S.H. (1985). Chronic pain: conceptualisation and epidemiology. Annals of Behavioural Medicine, 7, 3, 3–5.

Schuler, M. (1982). Sexual counselling for the spinal cord injured: a review of five programmes. *Journal of Sexual and Marital Therapy, 8*, 241–252.

Seligman, M.E.P. (1975). *Helplessness: On Depression, Development and Death*. San Francisco: Freeman.

Shadish, W.R., Hickman, D. and Arrick, M.C. (1981). Psychological problems of spinal cord injury patients: emotional distress as a function of time and locus of control. *Journal of Consulting and Clinical Psychology, 49*, 2, 297.

Shontz, F.C. (1975). *The Psychological Aspects of Physical Illness and Disability*. New York: Macmillan.

Siosteen, A., Lundqvist, C. and Blomstrand, C. (1990). The quality of life of three functional spinal cord injury subgroups in a Swedish community. *Paraplegia, 28*, 476–488.

Sipski, M.L. and Alexander, C.J. (1997) *Sexual Function in People with Disability and Chronic Illness*. Gaithersburg, MD: Aspen Publishers.

Slade, P.D. (1982). Towards a functional analysis of anorexia nervosa and bulimia nervosa. *Journal of Experimental Psychology, 38*, 168–172.

Smith, B., Buckett, J.R., Hunter-Peckham, P., Keith, M.W. and Roscoe, D.D. (1987). An externally powered multichannel implantable stimulator for versatile control of paralysed muscle. *Transaction in Biomedical Engineering, 34*, 499–508.

Spinal Injuries Association (1992). *Annual Review*. London: Spinal Injuries Association.

Staas, W.E., Formal, C.S. and Gershkoff (1988). Rehabilitation of the spinal cord-injured patient. In J.A. DeLisa (Ed.) *Rehabilitation Medicine: Principles and Practice*. Philadelphia: J.B. Lippincott.

Stanton, A.L. and Dunkel-Schetter, C. (1991). Psychological adjustment to infertility: an overview of conceptual approaches. In Annette L. Stanton and Christine Dunkel-Schetter (Eds) *Infertility: Perspectives from Stress and Coping Research*. New York: Plenum.

Stover, S.L. and Fine, P.R. (1986). *Spinal Cord Injury: The Facts and Figures*. Birmingham, AL: University of Alabama.

Swain, J., Finkelstein, V., French, S. and Oliver, M. (Eds) (1994). *Disabling Barriers – Enabling Environments*. London: Sage Publications.

Tennant, A. (1997). Models of disability: a critical perspective. *Disability and Rehabilitation, 19*, 478–479.

Tennen, H., Affleck, G. and Mendola, R. (1991). Causal explanations for infertility. In Annette L. Stanton and Christine Dunkel-Schetter (Eds) Infertility: *Perspectives from Stress and Coping Research*. New York: Plenum.

Trieschmann, R.B. (1986). The psychological adjustment to spinal cord injury. In R.F. Bloch and M. Basbaum (Eds.) *Management of Spinal Cord Injuries*. Baltimore, MD: Williams and Wilkins.

Trieschmann, R. (1987). *Aging with a disability*. New York: Demos.

Trieschmann, R.B. (1992). Psychosocial research in spinal cord injuries: the state of the art. *Paraplegia, 30*, 58–60.

Vasey, S. (1996). The experience of care. In G. Hales (Ed.) *Beyond Disability: Towards an enabling society*. London: Sage Publications, pp. 82–87.

Wade, D.T. and Langton-Hewer, R. (1987). Epidemiology of some neurological diseases with special reference to workload on the NHS. *International Rehabilitation Medicine, 8*, 129–137.

Wagner Anke, A.G., Stenehjem, A.E. and Kvalvik Stanghelle, J. (1995). Pain and quality of life within 2 years of spinal cord injury. *Paraplegia, 33*, 555–559.

Ward, A.B. and Houston, A.H. (1993). *Advice To Purchasers: Setting NHS Contracts For Rehabilitation Medicine*. London: British Society of Rehabilitation Medicine.

Weiner, B. (1979). A theory of motivation for some classroom experiences. *Journal of Educational Psychology, 71*, 3–25.

Weller, D.J. and Miller, P.M. (1977). Emotional reactions of patients, family, and staff in acute care period of spinal cord injury. *Social Work and Health Care, 3*, 1, 7–17.

Whalley Hammel, K. (1995). *Spinal Cord Injury Rehabilitation*. London: Chapman & Hall.

Whiteneck, G.G. (1989). Long term outlook for persons with high quadriplegia. In G.G. Whiteneck, C. Adler and R.E. Carter (Eds) *The Management of High Quadriplegia*. New York: Demos.

Whiteneck, G.G. (1990). The high costs of high-level quadriplegia. In D.F. Apple and L.M. Hudson (Eds) *Spinal Cord Injury: The Model*. Atlanta, GA: Shepherd Center for Treatment of Spinal Injuries, pp. 114–117.

Whiteneck, G.G., Carter, R.E., Charlifue, S.W., Hall, K.M., Menter, R.R., Wilkerson, M.A. and Wilmott, C.B. (1985). *A Collaborative Study in High Quadriplegia*. Englewood, CO: Rocky Mountain Regional SI System, Craig Hospital.

Whiteneck, G.G., Charlifue, S.W., Frankel, H.L., Fraser, M.H., Gardner, B.P., Gerhart, K.A., Krishnan, K.R., Menter, R.R., Nuseibeh, I., Short, D.J. and Silver, J.R. (1992). Mortality, morbidity, and psychosocial outcomes of persons spinal cord injured more than 20 years ago. *Paraplegia, 30*, 617–630.

Whiteneck, G.G., Charlifue, S.W., Gerhart, K., *et al.* (Eds) (1993). *Aging with Spinal Cord Injury.* New York: Demos.

Wilmuth, M.E. (1987). Sexuality after spinal cord injury: a critical review. *Clinical Psychology Review, 7,* 389–412.

World Health Organization (1947). Constitution of the World Health Organization. *WHO Chronicles, 1,* 29.

World Health Organization (1980). *WHO International Classification of Impairments, Disabilities and Handicaps: A Manual of Classification Relating to the Consequences of Disease.* Geneva: World Health Organization.

Yarkony, G.M. (1992). Spinal cord injured women: sexuality, fertility and pregnancy. In P.J. Goldstein and B.J. Stern (Eds) *Neurological Disorders in Pregnancy,* 2nd Edition. New York: Futura, pp. 203–222.

Yarkony, G.M., Bass, L.M., Keenan, V. and Meyer, P.R. (1985). Contractures complicating spinal cord injury: incidence and comparison between spinal cord centres and general hospital acute care. *Paraplegia, 23, 265–271.*

Yarkony, G.M., Roth, E.J., Heinmann, A.W., Yeongchi, W., Katz, R.T. and Lovell, L. (1987). Benefits of rehabilitation for traumatic spinal cord injury: multivariate analysis in 711 patients. *Archives of Neurology, 44,* 93–96.

Yarkony, G.M., Roth, E.J., Lovell, L., Heinemann, A., Katz, R.T. and Yeongchi, W. (1988a). Rehabilitation outcomes in complete C5 quadriplegia. *American Journal of Physical Medicine and Rehabilitation, 40,* 73–76.

Yarkony, G.M., Roth, E.J., Heinemann, A.W. and Lovell, L. (1988b). Rehabilitation outcomes in C6 tetraplegia. *Paraplegia, 26,* 177–185.

Yarkony, G.M., Roth, E.J., Heinemann, A.W., Lovell, L. and Yeongchi, W. (1988c). Functional skills after spinal cord injury rehabilitation: three year longitudinal follow-up. *Archives of Physical Medicine and Rehabilitation. 69,* 111–114.

Yarkony, G.M., Roth, E.J., Heinemann, A.W. and Lovell, L. (1988d). Spinal cord injury rehabilitation outcome: the impact of age. *Journal of Clinical Epidemiology, 41,* 173–177.

Yarkoney, G.M., Chen, D., Palmer, J., Roth, E.J., Rayner, S. and Lovell, L. (1995). Management of impotence due to spinal cord injury using low dose papaverine. *Paraplegia, 33,* 77–79.

Yeo, J.D. (1993). Prevention of spinal cord injuries in an Australian study (New South Wales). *Paraplegia, 31,* 759–763.

Zubek, J.P. (1969). *Sensory Deprivation: Fifteen Years of Research.* New York: Appleton Century Crofts.

Zuckerman, M. (1979). Attribution of success and failure revisited or: the motivational bias is alive and well in attribution theory. *Journal of Personality, 47,* 245–247.

Zwerner, J. (1982) Yes we have troubles but nobody's listening: sexual issues of women with spinal cord injury. *Sexuality and Disability, 5,* 3, 158–171.

Index